616.831

What you hear is not what you see : Alzheimer's, the second victim / by Cassandra Fleet.

Dec 2006

32487008759483
NEWARK PUBLIC LIBRARY-NEWARK, OHIO 43055

WITHDRAWN

What You Hear Is Not What You See

Alzheimer's The Second Victim

by Cassandra Fleet

American Literary Press
Five Star Special Edition
Baltimore, Maryland

WHAT YOU HEAR IS NOT WHAT YOU SEE

Copyright © 2006 Cassandra Fleet

All rights reserved under International and Pan-American copyright conventions. No part of this book may be reproduced, stored in a retrieval system, or transmitted in any form, electronic, mechanical, or other means, now known or hereafter invented, without written permission of the publisher. Address all inquiries to the publisher.

Library of Congress
Cataloging-in-Publication Data
ISBN 1-56167-931-3

Library of Congress Card Catalog Number:
2006903088

The images and events in this book do not represent any specific individual, living or dead.

Published by

American Literary Press
Five Star Special Edition
8019 Belair Road, Suite 10
Baltimore, Maryland 21236

Manufactured in the United States of America

Acknowledgments

I dedicate this book to my family, and all the families and their loved ones that I have cared for in the past.

Additional acknowledgment goes to my son-in-law William L. Fisher for his contributions and hard work in getting this book to press.

CONTENTS

WHAT YOU HEAR IS NOT WHAT YOU SEE	1
FAMILIES	3
THE GIFT OF GAB	11
THE WANDERER	21
SISTER	25
REPEATERS	35
WHAT TIME IS IT?	39
A DAY IN THE BATHROOM	43
THE POOP SMEARING	49
THE TEN-MINUTE PATIENT	53
NOW THAT'S A LITTLE SHOCKER	57
GUILT	59
DO YOU KNOW	65
ILLUSTRATIONS	68

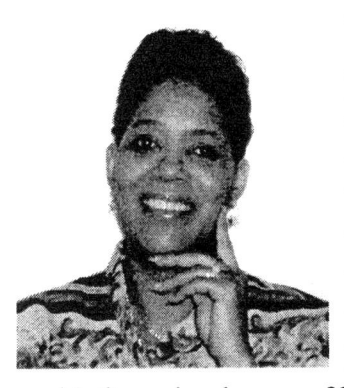

TWENTY YEARS AGO I had a friend who was a caregiver. Her client was a friend of mine as well. My friend fell sick and went to the hospital for a short stay. Well, I tried to be a good friend and cared for her client while she was ill. A few months later, my friend passed away and left me in charge of her client. By having the experience working with clients, in and out of nursing homes, day cares, and as a home care provider, I thought my experience would be enough. Well, I didn't know the half of it. I went from a wife and mother to a caregiver. As a wife I chose to get married and as a mother I knew that the sound of little feet was a part of me, but to wake up one day to an eighty-year-old man who didn't have family or anyone to call his own but me. This was a scary proposition to settle in my mind. To be responsible for an eighty-year-old adult will make you stop and think: **What have I gotten myself into?** I found myself crying a lot because there was no free time for my family, my husband or myself. I went from a parent with four kids to having five kids, with the oldest kid, eighty years old, needing to be changed, fed, washed daily, and watched twenty- four hours a day just to keep him safe. The trips to the doctor's office used all of my free time. I was overwhelmed with grief, to a point, and one step from seeing a doctor for my sanity. So in the interest of my well-being, I put my friend's client in a nursing home, and three months later he passed away. That's when a disturbing thought came to my mind: **Did I do the right thing?** The differences between my situation now and my first caregiving experience are: 1.) I care for my mother and brother, who is schizophrenic; 2.) I am the proud owner of an assisted living home with three hallucinating schizophrenic people living there; and 3.) helping one of my daughters cope with brain cancer—then I go home.

INTRODUCTION

Hi! My name is Connie and I have a love for old people. It started when I was five years old, back in 1953. When families kept their elderly family members at home and funerals were held in the living room. I had always thought that "as children we were blessed," because we knew so many old people, 60 to 90 years old. I got a chance to talk and walk with history. What I learned at five was old people get wrinkled as a prune, their skin as soft as cotton, and their memory is shot. Not all old people develop Alzheimer's. Some just have old age disease.

Now I'm known as "sir," a professional "poop cleaner." I've been one for twenty-five years. I want to share some of my short stories with you. It will help you to get through one day at a time with a sick person. I know that you cry a lot, and "cuss" a lot. You feel hurt a lot, and sometimes just want to give up.

I want you to laugh a lot. Think about it. Some of the things you see and hear are unbelievable. I want to refresh your memory. The first few months you think you have it good. Well, the honeymoon is over. Hello! You have someone in your home that is no longer your mother, father, brother or sister. They are like no one that you would want to care for and this is Shock Time! They belong to you, believe it or not.

WHAT YOU HEAR IS NOT WHAT YOU SEE

Imagine going to work, as a care giver, every day and a client calls you "Mister." I know that I stand 6 ft. tall, a teasing tan, short curly hair and a mother of three. To my clients, I am known as the "big man" or the "controller," the "teacher," the "boss" and the "sissy man."

People that work in this type of business have become accustom to clients that don't know if you are a man or a woman. What clients hear is the voice of authority. I find that it works in my best interest. The sounds they hear can be something from the past, like a grandmother or a father figure, but it works for me to keep the clients in control and safe. Again, just imagine going to work every day and be called Frank, Joe, Donald, Bill or even James. I think this would upset most of us, but not me. I am used to it now, most of the time. I am called "sir" and I think this name will stick with me for a long time. I have never heard my own voice before, but others have. I remember going to a clothing store and trying on a dress and shouting out, "This dress is too big," and clearing out the entire dressing room, because they thought a man was in the fitting room. On the telephone, I am constantly addressed as "sir" even if I spell my name to the operator. It just doesn't work.

Just because you look like a movie star and sound like a man it let's you know that people don't really see you, but they hear you. So in this instance, patients are not alone, this is the way of the world.

FAMILIES

I was five, and my mother and stepfather were just getting married. My stepfather took my mother, sisters, brothers, and me home to meet his mother. She was ill and in a wheelchair, swollen from top to bottom. Crying softly, just enough for me to hear her behind the bedroom doors, she was in the front room of the house. It was dark and dreary, all alone to suffer in her pain. I opened the door to take a peek at her, and to my surprise a little old gray headed lady was sitting in a wheelchair. I walked over to her to introduce myself. "Hi, my name is Connie and what is your name?" I said excitedly. She said, "Mary!" "Well Mary, this is a good day. The sun is shinning and the children are playing on the front steps. 'Would you like to go outside?'", I said. She responded, "Yes I would, but I can not walk." I looked down at her feet and they were swollen, as big as a baseball. I was not afraid, just a little surprised. I sat down on the floor and I held her foot in my lap and gently started to rub it softly. The touch of her foot was very hard. I was afraid I might hurt her. I looked up at her face and saw a smile that was soft as if I was rubbing her heart. I saw the sun come into that room as if God had opened the heaven. At that very moment, I believed that was my calling. My heart opened up to this little old woman with cancer, and I saw my kindness soothe her pain. It was like I had something no one else had, the gift to heal. For the next 50 years I found myself in places that only sick people would live; the nursing homes, community hospitals, state hospitals, and in their own homes. I knew then that my life would take me to this point. I have a love for the sick and homeless people in the world.

I have friends that are sick. Some have brain injuries and can't remember a thing, but in a glimmer of light comes happiness and a smile. If you catch it, at that moment, you will be overwhelmed with joy. God gives us all a brain to think, and when it stops remembering and thinking, we think all is lost; but on days like this, you just want to holler to someone telling them he smiled at me, or I just made a mistake. No, this is not a mistake. It's just to let you know they we alive. Just take one day at a time and rejoice in it, because tomorrow it may be all gone. What happened, and why it happened, and will it happen again, no one knows. Don't give up just be grateful for every day.

You know, sometimes they fight you, and you want to strike back, but you can't. They might be someone's mother, father, sister, or your family member. It's hard to keep focused on the job at hand. We call this "burnout." Now what should you do — go out and come in again, or step back, count to ten, breathe. Who knows what is good for a person working so closely with the sick person, not just with people with Alzheimer's or dementia disease, but with all kinds of diseases. We are only human, not a super hero; even if you want to be one.

What You Hear Is Not What You See

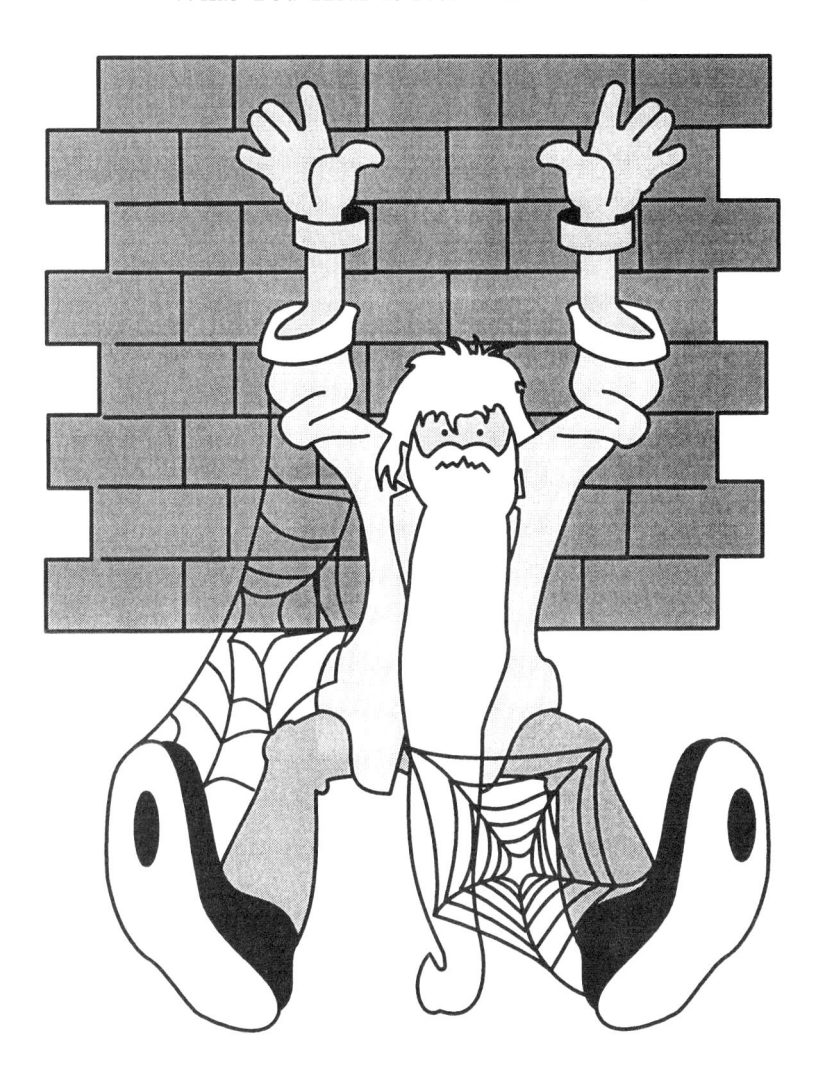

Citizen

Connie

"How can you prove that you are a citizen of the United States?"

Bill

"I'm not in jail."

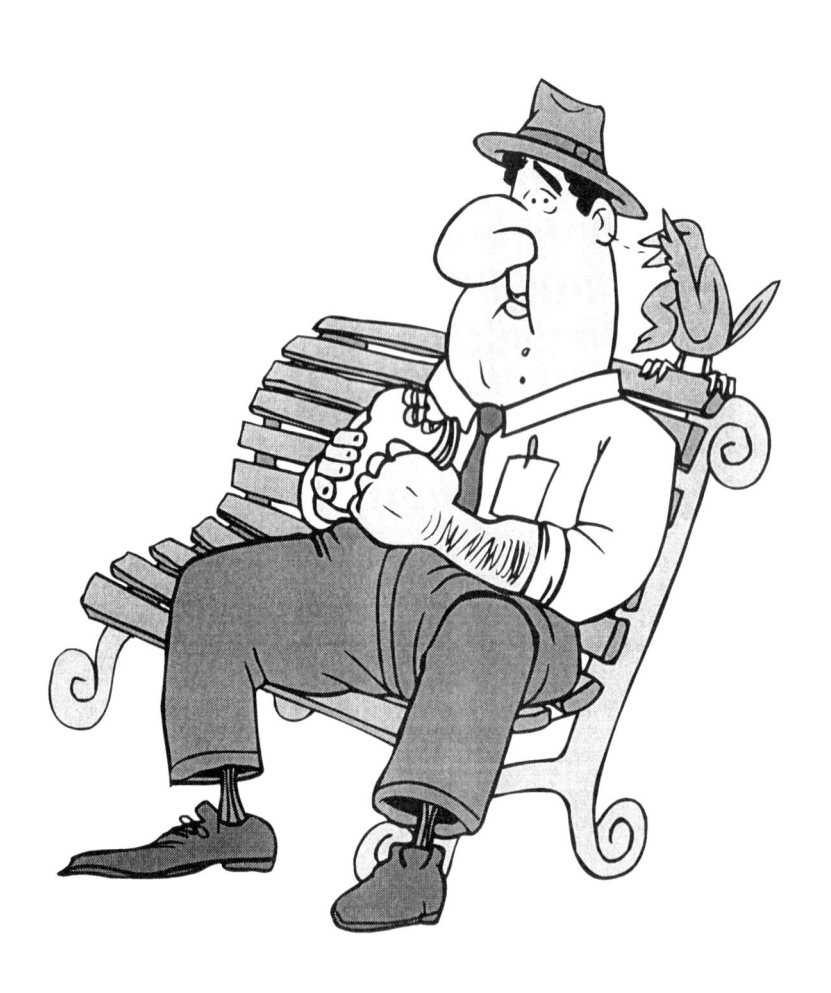

"Someone stole my car keys."

What You Hear Is Not What You See

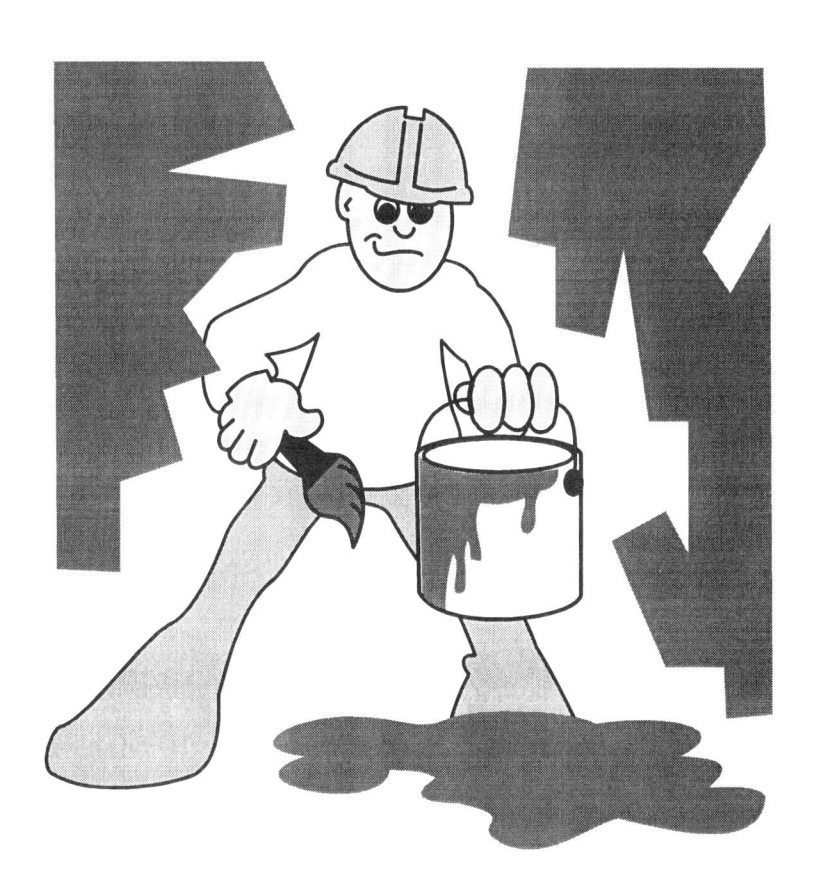

Art Class

Connie

"STOP!
Don't drink that.
It's paint."

Bill

"It's OK.
I like it.
It's pretty."

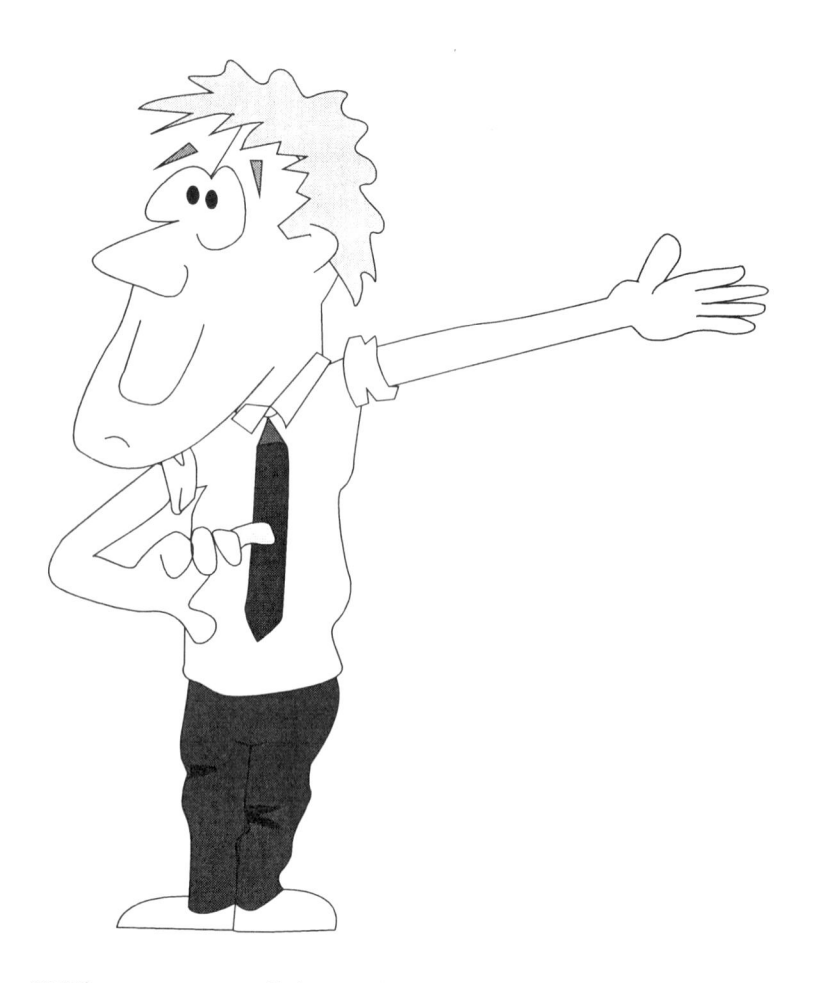

"Who are you talking to?"

"The people in the corner."

What You Hear Is Not What You See

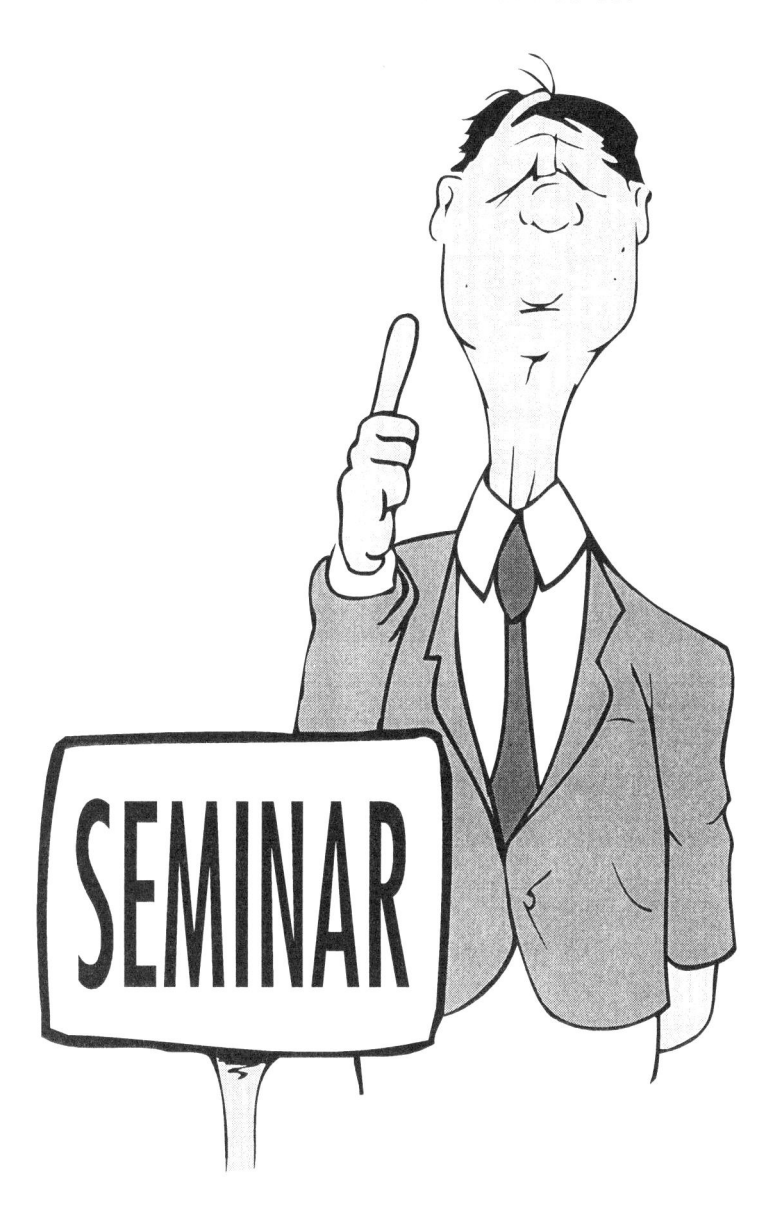

"What are you doing?"

"Reading to the people outside."

THE GIFT OF GAB

You need to learn the gift of gab. If they want to go, and you say "no," you got a fight on your hands. Well, there are tricks to this trade that would help you get out of it without anyone getting injured.

There are certain types of tricks that you can use on an Alzheimer's patient. It will amaze you to see how easy they are to do. I was sitting in the support group one morning and there was this lady and she was crying and crying! So, it was her turn to tell us her story. You know that personal story that nobody is supposed to know. She was crying up a storm. Well, her husband worked at Sparrows Point and his daily routine was to get up at 3 in the morning, get himself together, get his lunch, kiss his wife, and go to work. Well, he's been retired now for quite a while. Guess what! In his mind he still goes to work. This lady says that every morning, Monday through Sunday, he gets up and tears up her refrigerator. He's looking for his car keys and he's screaming and hollering, "I got to go to work. 'It's almost 4 a.m.'" He doesn't even know how to drive, and now this guy wants to get into a car and go to work. Well, he's been sick for a long time, but he would go outside and he would look around for the car. He'd do anything just to get to work. She didn't know how to stop him. Now she has to stop and think how to get Henry back in the house in bed.

First of all, Henry never did put clothes on. He was walking around in a pair of pajamas. Then she said, "Well Henry, let's go in the house and look for the keys." Henry didn't want to do that either. Henry had to go to work. "I gotta go to work", he would tell her. Then she said, "Well Henry, come in the house and let me make your breakfast for you." Henry would stop for a moment. He'd calm down just for a second and he'd say, "Okay, let me go get my lunch. I need my lunch." Then they would go back in the house. Once she got him in the house, she could lock the door again.

Now he's in the house and he still has to go to work. She is about ready to pull her hair out of her head. She doesn't know how to use the gift of gab. Now she's trying to talk to him in a low tone, "Come on sweetheart. Come on, let's go to bed. It's not time for you to go to work. It's just not time. Give it another hour." She would do anything that she could to try to get him upstairs. Well, Henry's calm and he goes back upstairs. It might work one time, but you'd better rest assured, tonight or tomorrow Henry is going to work again.

If she had used "the gift of gab" on Henry, she would have said something like, "Okay Henry, you're going to work. Let me go get your shoes for you. Okay, let me get your pants for you. What color socks would you like to wear, Henry?" There are a lot of things that you could say to change his mind. Once he looked at himself, he probably wouldn't have known he had on pajamas, because it wouldn't make any difference to him anyway. She could have said something like, "Okay Henry. I forgot your lunch. Let's go in the house and get your lunch." Once you got Henry in the house and you found a new way to lock the door, Henry couldn't get out for the second time. Seat him at the kitchen table and give him a sandwich. Ask him about his job. Ask him the types of things he used to do on his job. If he can remember, ask him when did he retire? How long did he work there? What are some of his buddies' names? Then you have to stop talking to Henry. See, you can't make him angry because then he would want to go to work again and it would be even harder to get him into bed. Now, while you are talking about all the good things with him, like his job, his coworkers, the years he's been on the job, and then you say, "Let me run you some bath water. Come on, you got to take a bath." Now you can get Henry upstairs. "Okay, let me lay you out some clothes." It sounds like a lot of work. True, it is a lot of work.

Now, I don't mean you actually have to run bath water. That's just something that you say to him to change his mind. See, anything that you say to Henry is going to last about three minutes. Okay, you are going to lay him out some clothes. Tell him to lie down for a minute until you cool the bath water off. Tell him the bath water was just a tad bit too hot. That's how you take control. He is going to lay down because he is tired from all of the jumping up he did last night. If he takes medicine, he doesn't have to know it. If you can't get his medicine in him, then give it to him in applesauce, Jell-O, or crush it or let him drink it, this will quiet him so he can rest. Most of the time, I find that they sleep the medicine off because they go to bed so early. I know if you're about 70 or 80 you don't want to stay awake until 10 or 11 o'clock at night. So you have to find ways to tire him out before you have "burnout." See, Henry has more energy than all of us put together. Henry knows he wants to go to work. He's going to fight you every step of the way. That's the hard part. Once you get Henry back upstairs and in bed, that's the easy part. You get the medicine in him, maybe Henry will go to sleep for the rest of the night and maybe you can get some rest too. What you need to do is learn the gift of gab and that is fast talking, changing minds and getting them redirected to where you need them to be.

What You Hear Is Not What You See

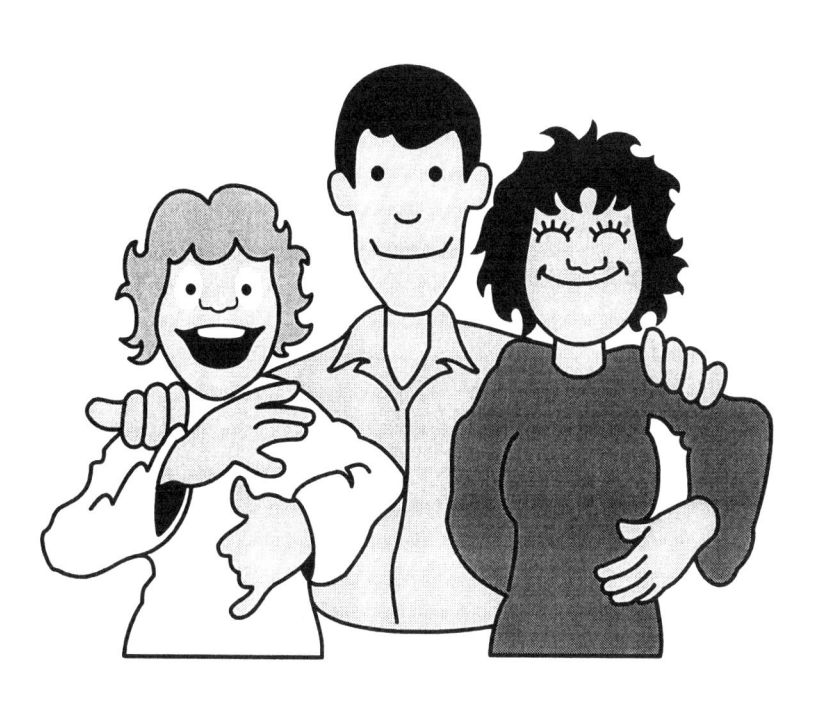

"Who are you kids?"

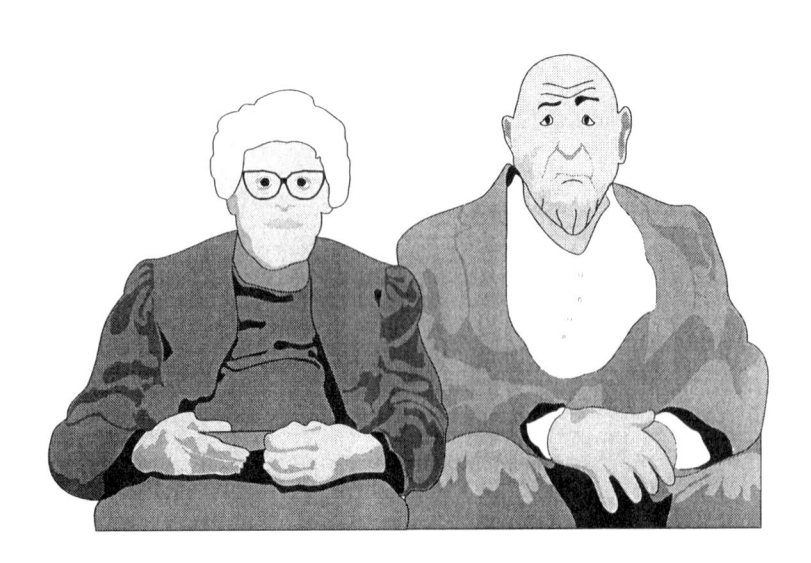

Maps

Connie

"Where is the
Pacific Ocean?"

Bill

"On left."

What You Hear Is Not What You See

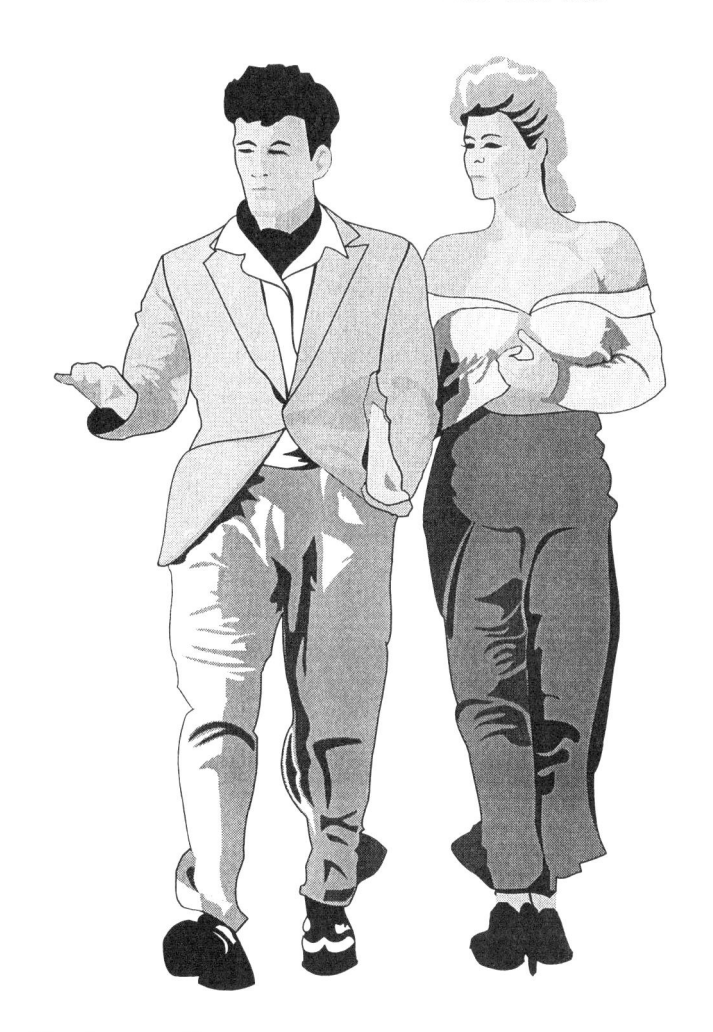

Trying to Remember

Bill

"I want my wife."

"No, not you, Fred, Mary!"

Connie

"I am here."

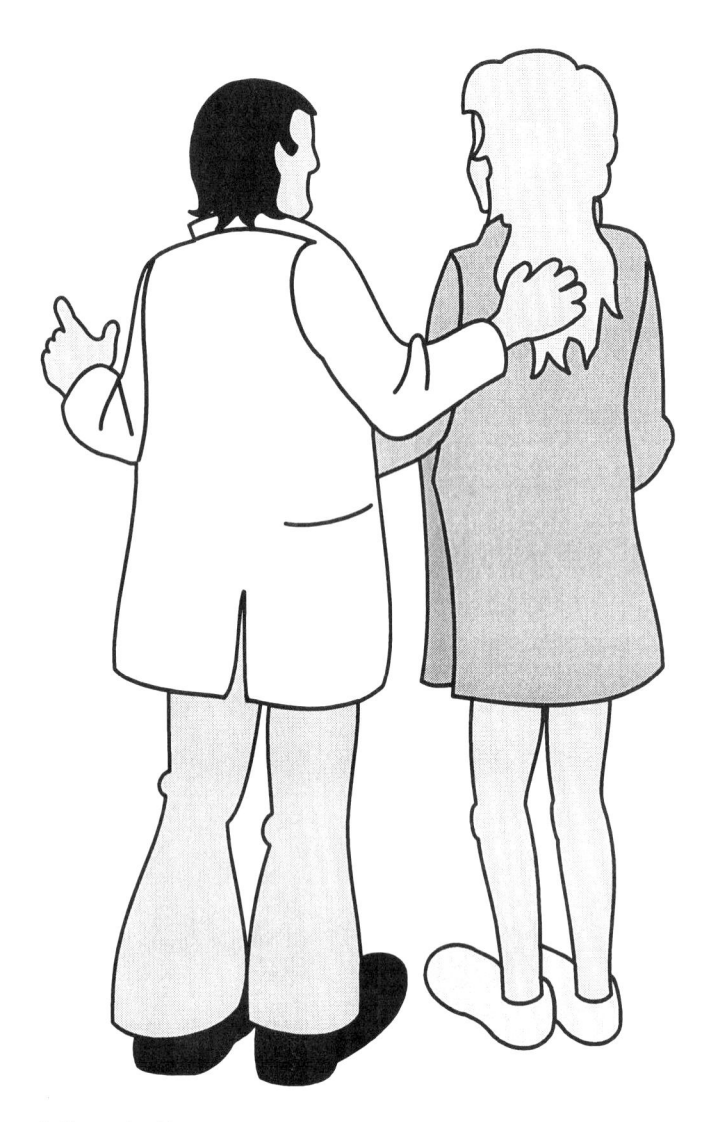

Married

Connie

"Daddy, how many children do you have?"

Bill

"None. I'm not married."

What You Hear Is Not What You See

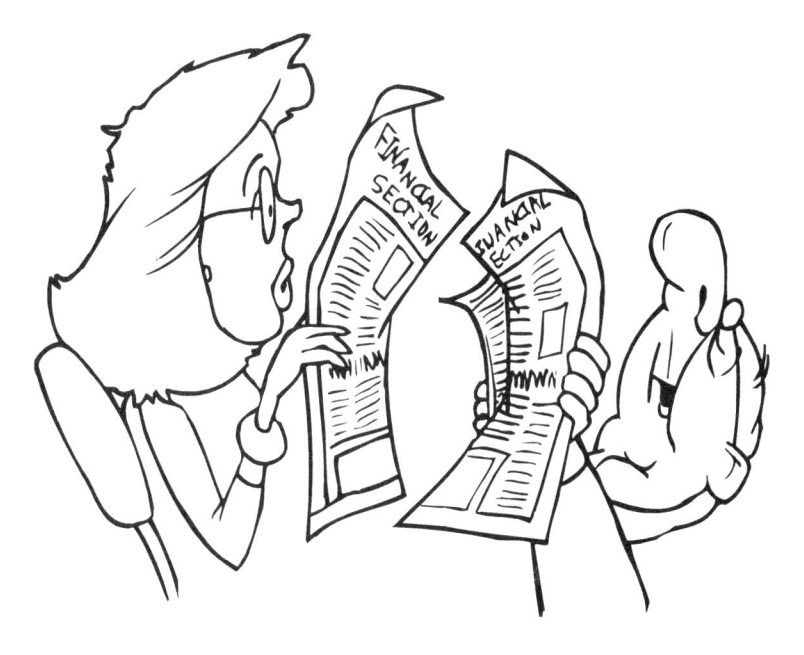

"Name the four seasons for me."

"Winter, spring, fall, and Halloween."

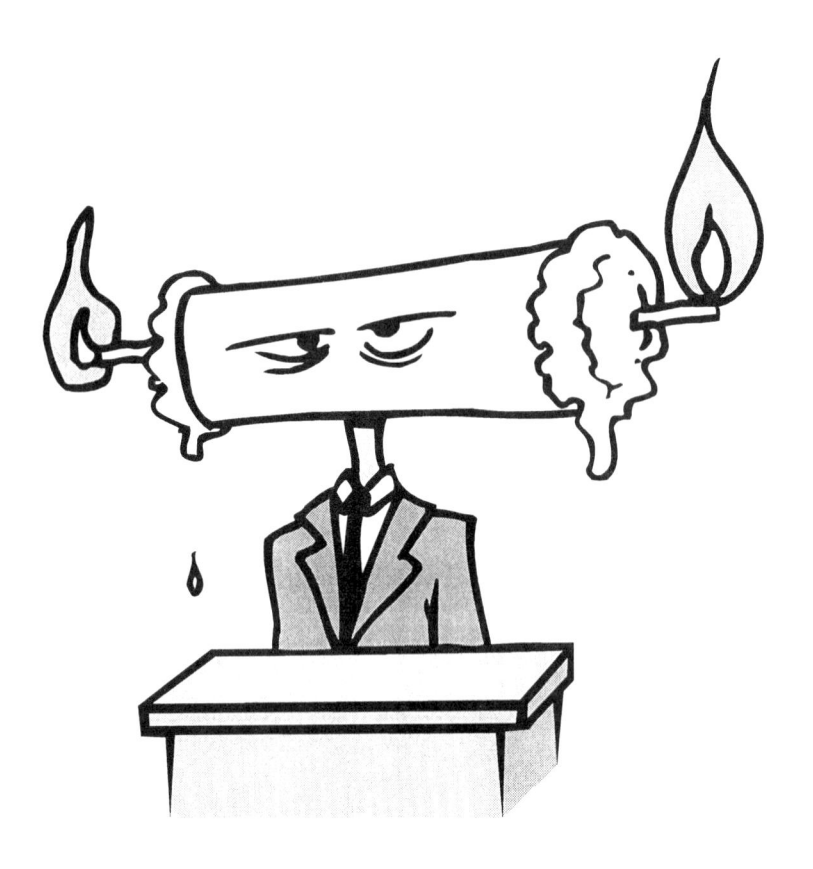

"Where are the matches?"

THE WANDERER

Some wanderers, like Henry, are constantly walking all day long, day in and day out. It could be some sort of reaction from the medications. You have to tire them out, so you can have time for yourself. Patients like him could walk 18 to 20 hours a day. This could drive you crazy and wear out your carpet, too. Sit down with them for maybe 5 or 10 minutes. See, we know that they're tired. Most of the time they're dehydrated and they're sweating themselves to death. You find that people that wander and walk a lot always lose a lot of weight. I don't care how much food you feed them, they will walk it off. You can even teach your children how to play these little "house games" with them.

    Start off with things like, "Can you whistle me a happy tune? Can you look in the mirror and make a funny face? Raise your left hand. Do you look at Sunday morning cartoons? Can you beat a drum? Do you like to dance? Who has on bright colors? Whose birthday is coming up?" These are some of the things that you can do with them.

    You can ask them to sing along with you. Do you like to listen to the radio? Ask them to tell you a little joke. Who likes Frosted Flakes cereal? You have to talk to them at least five to ten minutes until they calm down and change their mind.

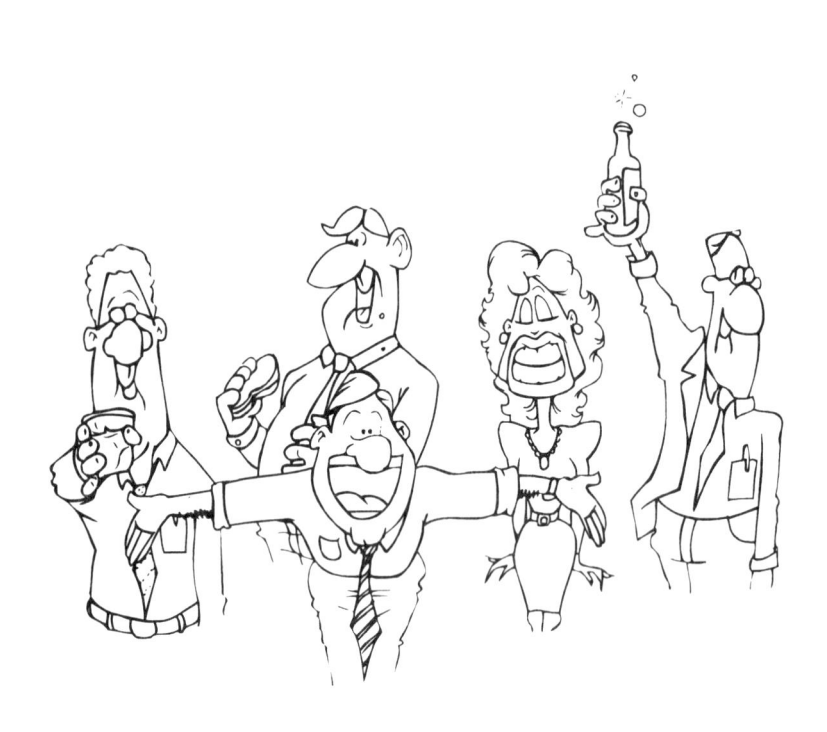

Happy Birthday

Connie

"Happy Birthday, Daddy. How old are you?"

"I thought you were seventy-two years old."

Bill

"Sixteen, and never been kissed."

"No, you don't know me."

What You Hear Is Not What You See

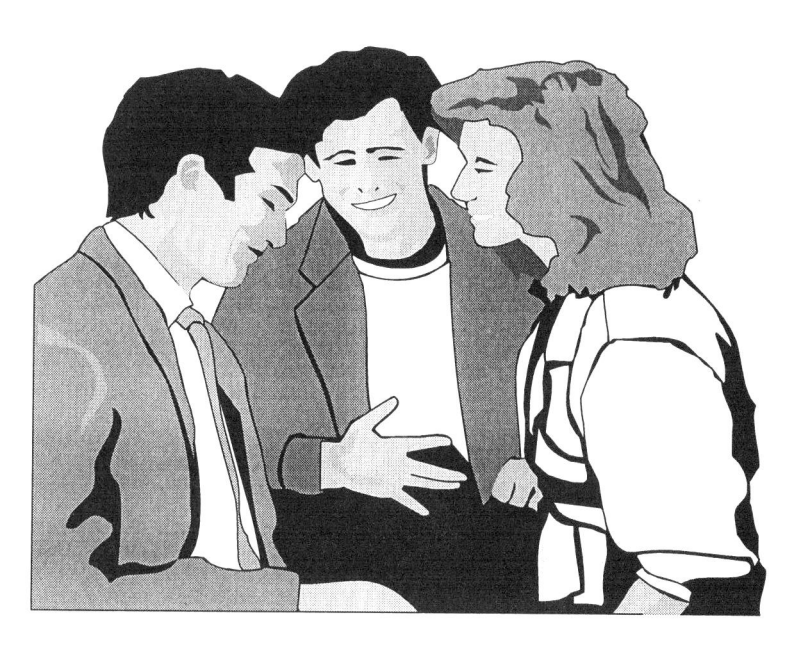

The Mail

Connie

"What is your zip code?"

Bill

"Bill, Jr."

SISTER

I was introduced to an older lady. Her name was Sue and she was 85 years old. She had a sister that was named Mary who was 84 and had Alzheimer's. I was told by Sue that Mary had not had a bath in eight months. Can you believe it? Eight months! Well, I thought she was really talking a little out of her head, but she invited me to come to Mary's house to see if I could give her a bath. Now, when I'm talking about the gift of gab, I've never used it so hard, so long and so seriously in my life.

When I got to Mary's house, I found that she was the type of person that wandered the streets. She collected people's mail; she collected their phone books. She went into people's cars and the neighbors were upset. Well Sue, 85 years old, couldn't do much with her 84 year-old-sister that had Alzheimer's, who would probably hit you in the blink of an eye. All Sue wanted was her sister to have a bath, and that was my job.

The first day that I met Mary, she had on about eight layers of clothes. It was shocking. The house had mail that was piled up to the ceiling. The kitchen had food piled to the ceiling. I tell you, it was so crowded in that house I didn't know where the front door was or how to get to the back door. All I knew, I was here to give Mary a bath. Well, looking through the house and going through things, I found that Mary used her entire house for a toilet. She used the bowl, tub, and the toilet but never flushed it. She used the kitchen, bedroom and anyplace else in the house as her bathroom. Before bathing Mary, I had to clean Mary's house. Once the house was clean, my job began. I had to get Mary out of eight layers of clothes, into the bathroom and give her a bath.

The entire time I was there, Mary was walking around with a broomstick in her hand. I had a cast on my left hand and I knew that she and I were going to fight somewhere or sometime during the day.

I would never hurt my patients, but I know my patients can sure enough hurt me if I give them a chance. I had to step back for a minute and think how I would approach her. I knew Mary was a wanderer. She would never sit down. She was always on the go and I knew I could never stand before her and talk with her. I had to think how I was going to get her in the bathroom.

The more I said, "Could you come in the bathroom, please". She would walk in the kitchen. I said again, "Can you come in the bathroom, please, I want to show you something" she would go out the front door. I actually had to lock us in the house. The funny part is I had to get rid of Mary's sister. I told her to go on the front porch and have a seat.

Now, Mary's sister is gone. The house is locked and it's time for me to switch roles with Mary. I am now Mary's mother or her enforcer. I know that sounds cruel, but now I am not asking Mary to come and take a bath, I am telling her it is time to take a bath. I grab Mary by

What You Hear Is Not What You See

the hand and with a little resistance I take her into the bathroom. I start to talk to her very softly, like, "Oh, we're going to be beautiful when I get finished. Oh, let me take this off. This dress is sort of dirty. Let me put something clean on you."

I showed Mary her clothes, slips and underwear. These items would appeal to most women. I showed her a pretty scarf for her head and a pretty pair of red shoes. Now Mary is interested in the shoes and began talking.

Now a conversation has changed to beautiful clothes, and beautiful red shoes and how about a pair of red earrings to match those shoes. I continued to bring her deeper into the conversation and say "Do you carry a pocketbook, Mary? and 'When is the last time that you've been to church?, and Do you like church?, and Can we sing a church hymn? Do you know one, Mary? Let's sing one.'" We proceed to sing church songs at the same time I am taking off eight layers of clothes from her body, while still talking about red shoes. The water in the tub is lukewarm. I didn't want it too hot.

Now you understand about the bathroom scene and how strange a bathroom looks to patients. I put a chair in the tub so Mary doesn't have to sit so far down. I also fill the tub with just above two feet of water; I didn't want her to become frightened believing she is going to drown. I now have Mary in the tub. I bathed her and washed her hair too.

See, I could tell from the style of Mary's clothes and how expensive they are that Mary, at one time, was a well-dressed lady. Also from the furniture in her house, I could tell she was also a "well-off" lady. Last but not least, I knew that Mary was the owner of five apartment buildings. I knew she was a woman of some character and I used her character to work her into the bathroom.

Now with this fast talking, Mary is in and out of the tub. She's now in front of a mirror. Even though she may not know it's her, Mary can see the clothes that I'm putting on her. Just remember, about 20 minutes earlier the stockings had been on her legs for eight months and I was pulling off her skin along with the stockings. Now I've greased her legs down and I'm putting on new stockings, new underclothes, new slip and a clean suit. Now Mary is starting to smile and she is looking good. Even though the lady in the mirror doesn't look like Mary, she knows whoever that woman is, she looks good to her.

We're still talking about church and things that I know that Mary used to do in her lifetime. This worked to my advantage. See, I used Mary's personality, again, to win her over. It was kind of hard at the beginning, but this is how you fast talk your patients. Using the gift of gab can change anybody's mind. This, with a normal person, would be called a "flimflam." A flimflammer can beat you out of your money, your house, your children, and anything else that they want. All by using fast talking to confuse the person who they are talking too.

Basically, that's what we're doing to our clients. It's not flimflam, but it's definitely fast talking. We have changed their minds so much, so fast, we confuse them, and we are able to get the job done. I stuck with Mary for quite a while until she had to eventually go into a nursing home. To my surprise, she went back to her sister, Sue.

I did not know the man that was on the porch waiting for us to give Mary a bath and get her house cleaned was Sue's husband. He had Alzheimer's too. I walked up to him to shake hands and say, "How do you do?" The gentleman pulled out a pear and said, "Hi, I'm saving this." The instant I looked at this guy and had a short conversation I realized that this poor lady, at 85, not only had a sister with Alzheimer's but a husband too. You know the shocking part about this story? She was 85 years old, couldn't walk too well and was in bad health. She allowed her husband, with Alzheimer's, to drive her around to take care of her sister.

I remember Sue telling me to come back to her home so that she could pay me for the job, and this gentleman got in the driver's seat. Well my God, I thought I would just scream bloody murder! I followed these two in my car because it was unbelievable that this lady had to use her husband, knowing that he was sick, to get her around to tend to her sister.She let him man drive! Well, I followed him for eight blocks. He went up the wrong street. I saw her motioning to him in the car in front of me, to turn around and go the other way. Can you imagine being in the car with an Alzheimer's patient driving that has no fear, no sense of direction, and couldn't hold a two minute conversation? Let me tell you, it got worse, and I was having a heart attack behind them while following him home. He hit an intersection and never stopped. For some reason they have a radar. Do you remember that you would have a dog and you thought the dog was lost, but the dog could always find its way back home? This man, sure enough, drove up to the front of his house, parked the car, and didn't know how to get out after he'd gotten there. The wife opens the door and tells him, "Come on, let's go to the house." I tell you, I had never seen anything like that in my life, butI can tell you, there's a secret behind every door and a story to be told.

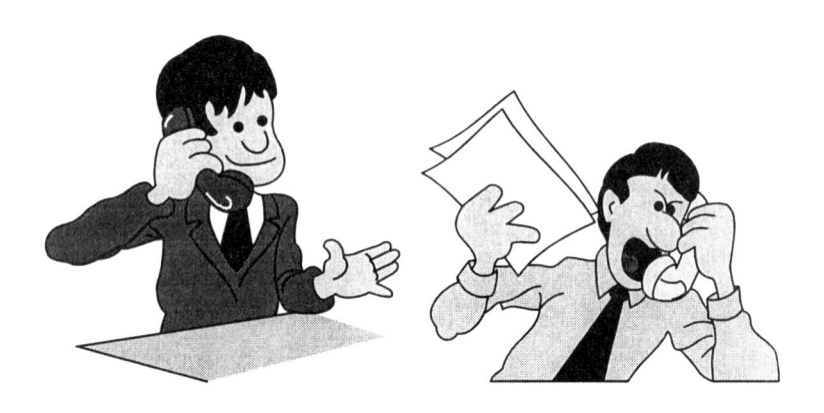

Telephone Ringing

"Hello, Bill.
Bill, is that you?"

"Hi.
No, it's me."

What You Hear Is Not What You See

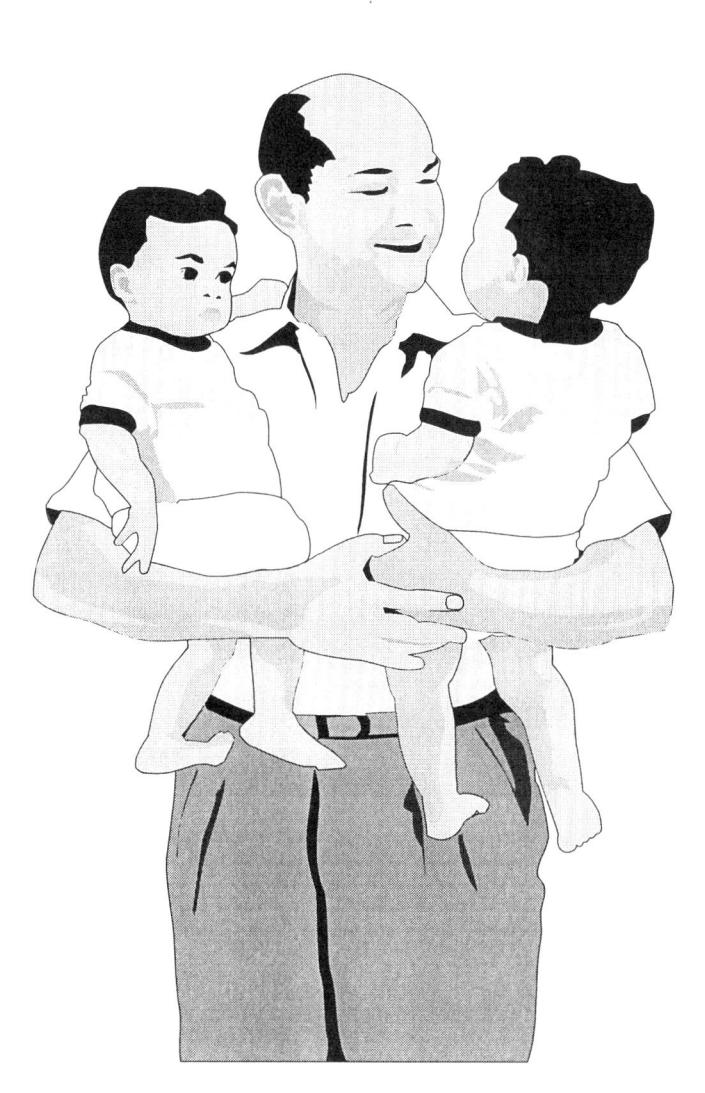

"I'm thirty-nine, not eighty-nine."

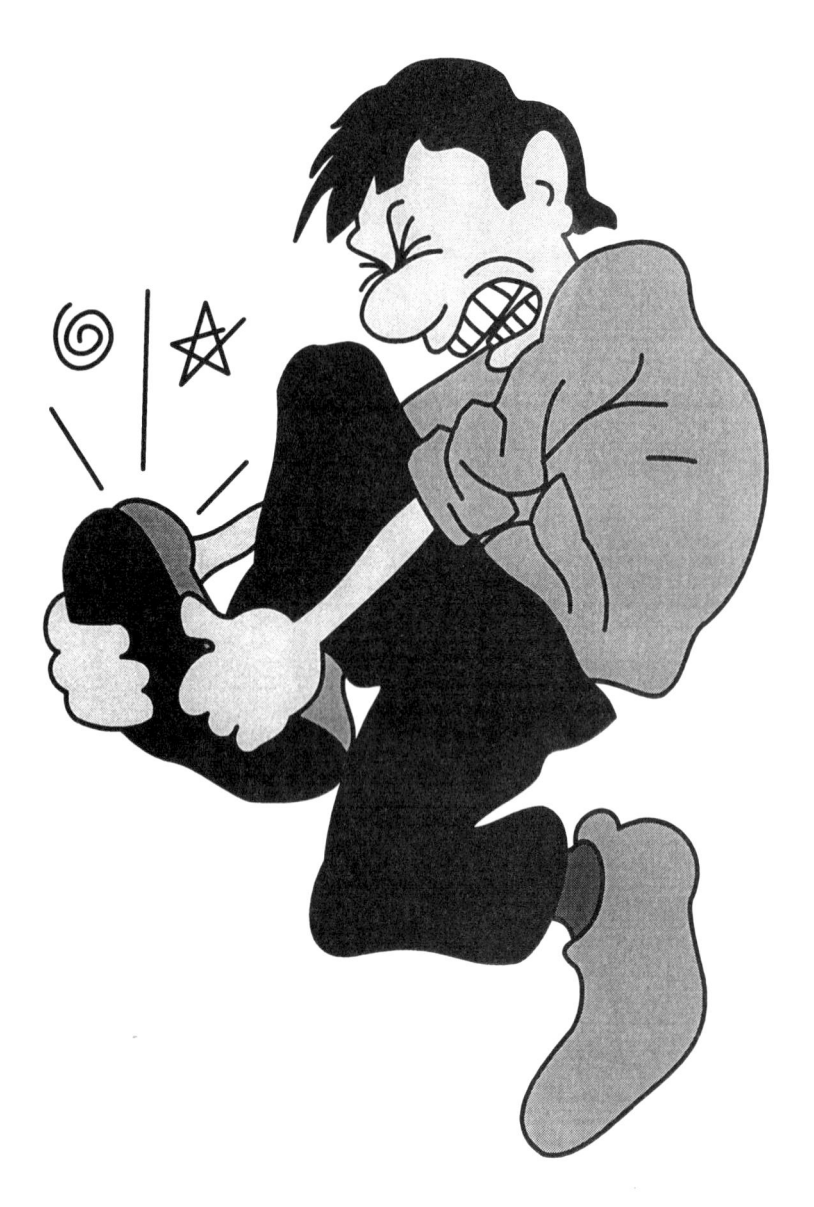

"I can't find my shoes. My feet hurt."

What You Hear Is Not What You See

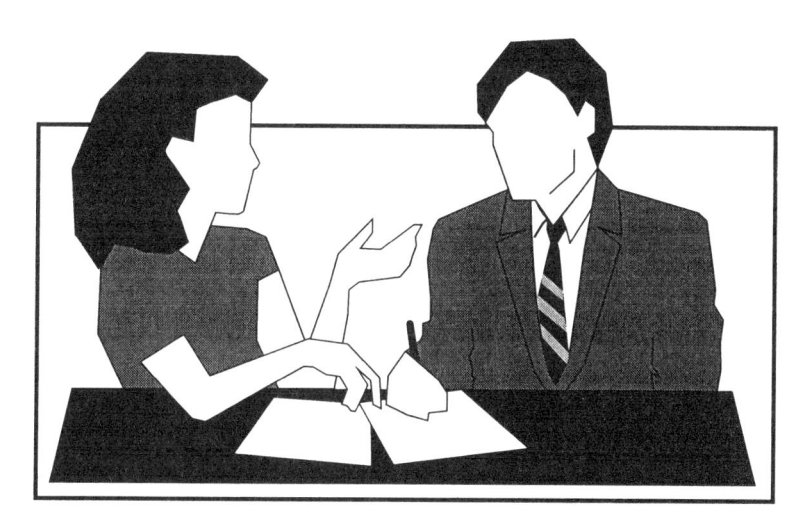

Your Name

Connie

"What is your name?"

Bill

"Thirty-nine."

REPEATERS

Yes, there are some people that the gift of gab, and nothing else, would work on. I find that working with many types of Alzheimer's patients on all different levels can be a job, no matter what you think you know. I mean, after 20 years of working with patients, you would think you had it down packed. It really isn't true, because every day there is something new for you to learn.

Some of the outpatients are — I call — repeaters. That means that every two minutes they come back and ask you the same question over and over again. It could be almost anything, like, "Are we ready to go home yet?" and you would tell them, "At 2 o'clock." Two minutes later, before they could sit down they say, "Are we ready to go home yet?", and then you would try to hold a conversation.

Now you're going to try to use the gift of gab on them, because they have asked you the same question about ten times a day and you're about ready to pull your hair out. You would say to them, "Where do you live? Do you have any children? Did you come here on the bus? Do you drive? Have you ever driven a car? Where did you work?" You think that's going to get their mind off the subject. You're asking them all of those questions and two minutes later you would say something like, "Okay, have a seat. At 2 o'clock we're going home." Well, low and behold, they turn around, walk 20 paces, return to their chair and go right back over to you again, "Are we ready to go home yet, because I'm getting tired".Well, they're back again. I mean these type of people would never give you a break, because from the time you see them in the morning, if they go to a daycare or at a nursing home, until the time they get there at seven in the morning and leave at 3 o'clock, they probably would have asked you that same question a hundred times or more.

You try to fast talk them and change their mind, but they have a one-track mind. They want to go home. Now, even if you took them out for a walk, or you said, "Okay, we're going home. Where do you live?" They know nothing but in their head they want to go home. Now some people or patients would say, "I live in Georgia". You know we are in Baltimore. "Well, I live in California and my mother's there too." They all want to go home. That means that there's nothing that you can say or do to change their minds.

What You Hear Is Not What You See

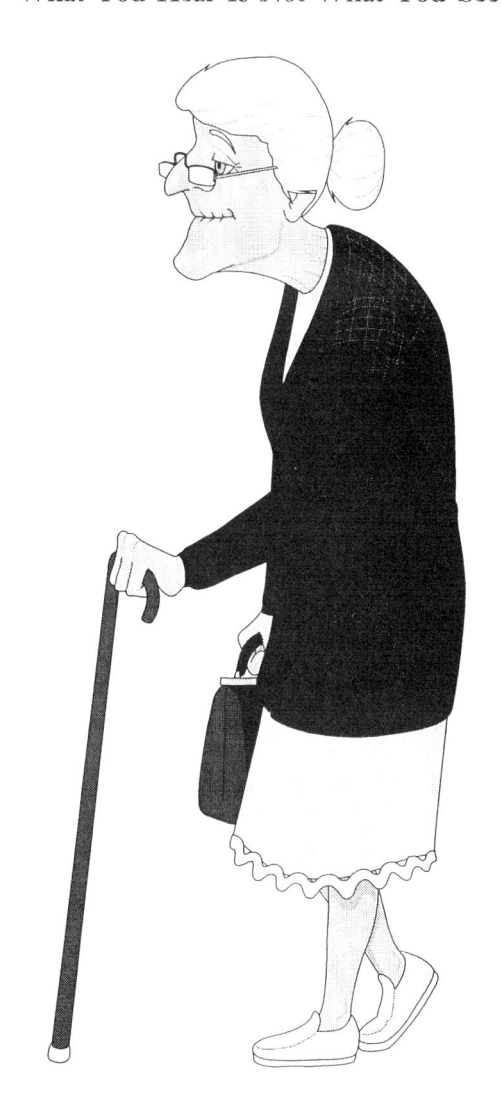

Cold Weather

Bill

"Mom, are you cold?"

Connie

"No, my hands hurt. I want to take it off."

WHAT TIME IS IT?

I had one lady who thought about "time" constantly. All day long she would say, "What time is it? What time is it?" I never understood why this lady always worried about the time, but I did find out later that she was in politics. I believe everything she did was due to time. You know how busy politicians are. Well, their day was scheduled out and this was the way the lady was. Everything she did was scheduled out. She had to know what time it was all day long. Just imagine, you are in the room with this lady and every five or ten minutes she wanted to know what time it was.

I had some patients that thought they had to go to the doctor's office everyday. Well, isn't a cab going to come and get me? I have a doctor's appointment. You would say, "Well, what day is your appointment? You are trying to fast talk them again and they say, "Today", and you say, "Well, what day?" They don't care what day. They just know that they have one right now, right at this moment. Well, that could go on all day long. Don't let them have a quarter in their pocket. They will want to use the telephone. "Can I call the cab? I have a doctor's appointment."

The more you say something like, "Well, we don't

have a public phone. We don't have a telephone", they will tell you, "Well, I heard one ringing. You are lying to me. I'm going to have you locked up." Now you have made them angry, because you were not talking fast enough to change their minds. Most likely you couldn't change their mind anyway, because they do this all day, every day.

Now you are about ready to go to jail because they want to call the police. They think you are holding them hostage. I'm telling you, it could drive you crazy. I don't know how I can keep my composure sometimes. Well, the day goes on and they're constantly asking you questions and you will actually find yourself sitting there trying to think of things to tell them or ask them so that you can change their mind.

Imagine walking around being one of those patients and you have one thing on your mind all day. Do you know that it could worry the patient to death? I've seen them break down and cry. "You just don't hear me. You just don't understand. I have to go home or I have a doctor's appointment or I have to go. My mother's waiting for me, or my children are home waiting for me. I have to baby sit."

Now this lady or man could be 80 or 90 years old and have babies at home they have to watch. I'm telling you, the topics that come out of their mouths will have you trying to figure out what to tell them. It takes a lot out of you, and it definitely will take its toll on you at the end of the day. It can work your mind until you don't want to think about a thing.

If you are at home and your mother or husband asks you the same question all day, you can't get your housework done because they're right behind you saying, "I want to go home to my mother. I have a doctor's appointment" or anything, you just don't know what to do. From the time they open their eyes until the time they go to sleep they have a one-track mind. You can't fast talk them at all, and they're going to be time conscience day in and day out.

A DAY IN THE BATHROOM

I'd like to give you some information about a day in the bathroom with an Alzheimer's patient. It will sound kind of rough and outrageous, because people don't want to talk about it, but they know and I know that these are things that really happen. A day in the bathroom with an Alzheimer's patient is a day of horror for the caregiver.

Hello, it's time to take my patient to the bathroom and I know it won't be a pleasant job. For anyone who's never dealt with an Alzheimer's patient in the bathroom, this is going to sound very strange, but it is actually the truth.

There are a lot of things you shouldn't do when taking a patient to the bathroom. The first is, you should never let them stand over the toilet and then you flush it. What they see and you see are not the same thing. To them, this rushing water is probably them falling off a cliff. If they started screaming and you don't know why, you won't, if you have never been in a bathroom with an Alzheimer's patient. Alzheimer patients don't see or hear or relate to things the way they used to. What they see is just in their head, and that is a world all of their own. We are not patients like them and we can't get into their heads. We don't know what it's like, but by working with them one—on-one, day by day, night by night, minute-by-minute, you will find out the most amazing things.

When you are standing in the bathroom with an Alzheimer's patient and you say, "Oh, look in the mirror. "Who's that lady?", and she tells you, "Oh, who are those group of people?" She sees but she doesn't see the same thing you see. If she's standing over the toilet and you are flushing the toilet just to make sure it's clean, of course, she sees that water and you're going to tell her to sit down? You must be crazy! For one, the toilet isn't a toilet to her, because in my experience I find that the kitchen plate they just ate out of is a toilet. The scrub water in the kitchen is their toilet. The washbowl in the bathroom is a toilet. The tub in the bathroom is their toilet. The last thing they think about is the toilet. There's nothing special to them and nothing bothers them at all. It only bothers us.

You have to constantly keep your eye on them at all times because if you don't you will be horrified. Actually, their stool in the toilet does not bother them. You might look up one day and they're coming to you and saying, "Here, this is for you." You respond, "What, what it is?", and then you look in their hands and find their feces. Well, you are about to really scream bloody murder, and wonder how could they do something like that? It does not bother them. Trust me. When they see something in the toilet they just get it. They don't know what it is. Actually, they don't even know that they put it in there. When you say, "Go to the bathroom", they have no idea what that means. If it comes out of them it comes out of them. If you don't have a regulated bathroom routine, every two hours, you will be cleaning up mess from the front door to the back door. These people have forgotten what it means to "go to the bathroom."

Sometimes they can go to the bathroom, and they will sit in there for hours. If you don't go in there and get them, they will be in there until tomorrow morning. I've seen people go into the bathroom, sit there, and play with the toilet paper and everything else in there. Have you ever heard one say, "Oh, there's Butch", and you want to know who's Butch? Well, Butch is an imaginary dog and they're sitting on the toilet talking to him.

"That's my dog", and you'll say, "Describe him for me." They could tell you in detail what Butch looks like, but they have no idea that they're sitting on the toilet to have a bowel movement, wipe themselves, wash their hands, get up, and leave. It means nothing to them. But they do see a dog. There's one thing about an Alzheimer's patient you should always know, they are never wrong. Everything they see, everything they do, you are still to say, "It's okay." That's hard to do when you're used to saying, "That's not right. That's not the way you do things. That makes no sense. This is crazy and that is crazy." To them everything is okay. Don't ever, ever, try telling them, "Butch is not in the bathroom" or "You need to make a bowel movement in the toilet." That doesn't work for them. You have to use a little strategy. This is why I say again, you must go to school, workshops, you must research, and you must be taught that there's a lot of things you would normally do that is no longer normal to an Alzheimer's patient. You know, naturally, we would know when we have to go to the bathroom, but being an Alzheimer's patient and having some brain defects, "knowing" and "going" doesn't do it. I've seen patients in nursing homes that would probably frighten the average person to death. They are called "the pickers", and I don't mean picking cotton or picking beans or plucking tomatoes or peaches off of a tree. I mean a "poop picker." The "poop picker" can sit in a bed in a nursing home; you can give them coffee, oatmeal, and a piece of toast and they can sit there for a minute. They can eat normally, like you and I would. The instant that they're finished, the next think you know, you come to get their tray and what's in the bowl where the cereal used to be - poop. The "poop picker" can lie in that bed under the cover and put their legs up or turn to the side. They can go up in their little butts and pick poop forever. I know it sounds kind of terrible, but this is actually the truth. These are things that you never talk about. It would never come out of your house because I'm sure there are some of us that have one "poop picker' in the home.

What You Hear Is Not What You See

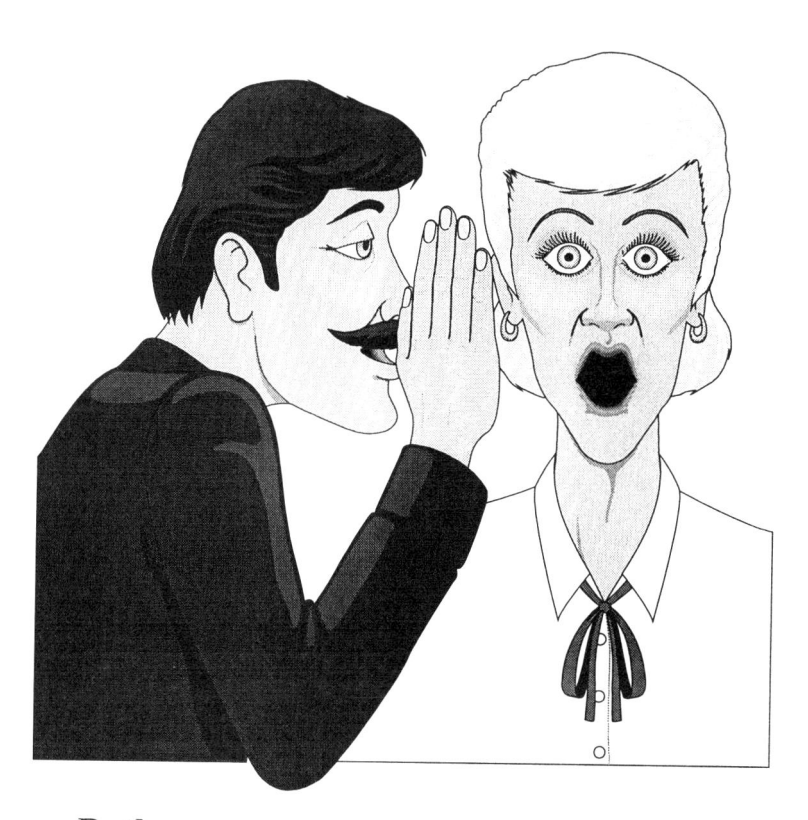

Bathroom

Bill

"Connie, do you need to go?"

Connie

"Go where?"

THE POOP SMEARING

Okay, I have told you about the "poop picker". Let's talk about those that do the smearing. Oh God, now what is a smearer? A smearer is one of those you give an Ex-Lax, Correctol to everyday, to keep their bowels a little loose. You know that you have to regulate their bathroom hours to every two hours; at least that's what you think. Those people that are smearers will go into the bathroom, take one square of that toilet paper, split that in half, wipe themselves three times and then smear feces along the walls, the rails, and the toilet. If you say, "Come on, you're finished?", they'll smear it on you too. That's the smearer. When they come out of the bathroom, they have it down their legs and on the back of their shoes or socks. They smear mess from the bathroom door to the bedroom down the hallway, down the steps and all the way to the kitchen. All you know is that the house smells like an outhouse, and an outhouse is what it is. It's mess everywhere. I'm telling you, you must keep your eye on them every minute of the day. That sounds hard, but if you have a routine or if someone can do shifts with you, your job isn't one times harder. They don't do it on purpose. They are doing the best that they can. You don't tell your mother, "Go upstairs and go to the bathroom, Honey, because I know you have to go." If you don't watch her go upstairs and you don't watch her go into that bathroom and sit down on that toilet, the lady could go out the front door and be reported missing for three or four days. Now you're in a panic because this week she went to the bathroom. Another week later, you think she still can go? Alzheimer's disease can move to a new level on them so easily, if you're not watching. You didn't study, you didn't do your homework and you didn't know that last week she could go to the bathroom by herself, but this week, she cannot. So you're looking for your mother and she is on the highway. Now it's time for you to call the police and scream and holler and pray to the Lord that your mother hasn't been hit, kidnapped, raped, killed or lost without anyone to help her. When I say go to school, again, you must study. It's in your best interest to know what you can do to protect your family members.

You know what kills me about the bathroom situation? I'm going to blame it on the women this time. You know, you could have a baby and that baby doesn't get up and say, "Okay, Mommy" — that baby's only about four months old — "Mommy, I have to go to the bathroom." What does the baby do? The baby might cry, or might be fidgety. I mean, there is a way you know that this baby is either wet or had a bowel movement. You will instinctly know that your baby needs to be changed. Well, your parents are almost in the same situation. Some of our patients do little things that let you know that their stomach is tight and they need to go to the bathroom, but they don't remember, and they won't say

What You Hear Is Not What You See

it. If you look into their faces and they sort of frown for no reason at all or they hold their stomach and they are sort of leaning over, you can tell that something is wrong. Now your job steps in. You should check them. You should check their pamper, if they wear one. You should constantly ask them. Whether they say they do or they don't, your job shouldn't stop right there. If you're not sure, you take them to the bathroom anyway. What you should remember is the last time they went to the bathroom. What did they just eat? How much did they eat? You know, they are babies and we do have to switch the roles. They're not three or four months old. They're 80 and 90 years old, but they are still babies. You have to be alert at all times, at all costs to take care of this person, because what you don't know is if that bowel movement stays on them long enough, dry up hard enough, and happens regularly, they'll end up with an ulcer. You don't want to know what it's like to have an ulcer, or treat an ulcer. If you have seen or cared for someone with an ulcer you know what I'm talking about. When their skin start to break down because they're constantly wet or constantly wear poop on their butt, they will get a sore on their back that will turn into a hole. You don't see this hole getting any better. Not only that, now they have an ulcer and that's bad. You think you will be going to the bathroom every two hours? Hmm, you're going to be in the bathroom or changing their diaper every 20 minutes because then it's going to be a "prescription by the doctor" situation.

Cassandra Fleet

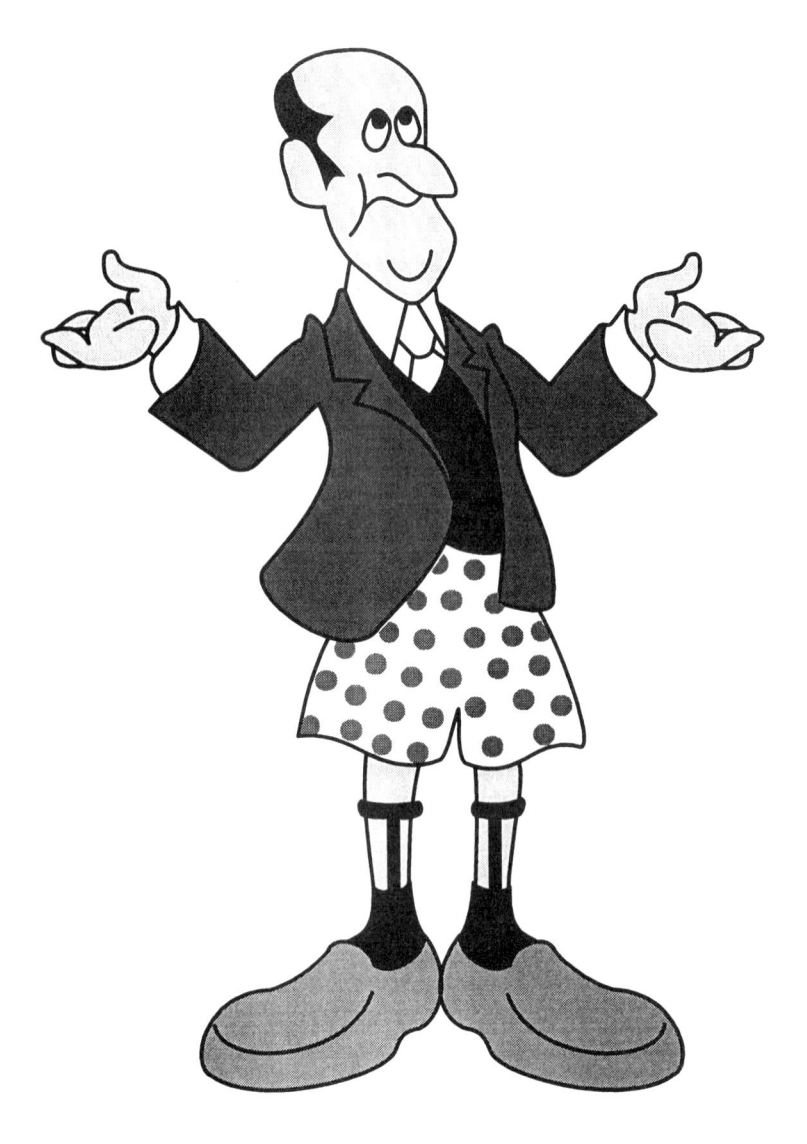

"Dad, where are you going?"

"To church."

"You can't walk there."

THE TEN-MINUTE PATIENT

I haven't told you about the "10 minute" man or woman. That's the person that goes to the bathroom, every 10 minutes, and you think that a person can't go to the bathroom every 10 minutes. Hah! You ought to see some of the Alzheimer's patients I've cared for in my house. I was doing "respite care" and this male client would have to go upstairs to the bathroom. Well, by the time he had gotten down the steps, and hit the living room door, he had made a U-turn and went back up the steps. Now remember you can't take your eyes off of him because if he's going up the steps and he has a slight problem walking and you're afraid that he might fall down the steps. Well, you can't tell him that he can't go and he doesn't know what you're talking about. When you say, "No," he thinks, "Go" and you are back upstairs in the bathroom. I have to follow them. That is a job in itself. I spend a day — just going back and forward to the bathroom. I constantly state, "Well, they go in the bathroom. They don't know what they're supposed to do. It's just a habit." They go in there and they sit down and they get up and they come right back out again, because the body is telling them to go. Well, believe it or not, those little minute people actually are going to the bathroom. I don't know what causes it, or how you could stop it, or anything else, but they're actually using the bathroom. If it's just a couple of little leaks, or maybe one little poop, it's okay. They really do have to go.

See, I told you in the beginning of this story that anything that an Alzheimer's patient does or says or whatever, it's okay. I know it's very tiresome for those that are up in age, but I think that it's hard for anybody of any age to care for someone. One day, I told a gentleman that he had been in the bathroom 20 minutes today and that I've been walking up and down for the last six hours. He said, "I have to go." I said, "No! You don't have to go." He said, "I have to go." Well, I was sorry that I said something like that. I saw it coming down his pants legs and into his shoes, in my living room, down the hall, up the stairs, and in the bathroom. He didn't even make it to the toilet. He sat on the side of the tub, and that's were it all fell out.

See, it's very hard to tell exactly what's going on in their heads. I think we really have to learn what's going on with the body. The body is a very delicate piece of machinery and if you fill it up, it's going to come out. That's the biggest problem. I had a good idea that I would regulate his food? Well, I would feed him a little lunch, I'd feed him a little dinner and I'd give him a nice breakfast with a glass of milk. Well, what I didn't know was, everybody cannot drink milk, or at least he couldn't. I would give him the milk and low and behold, the man would have diarrhea. He would have diarrhea for several days.

I continued to give this man milk and after about four days, I found out that this man would have a bowel movement every 20 minutes. That's why he continued to go to the bathroom. He didn't tell me, or he couldn't tell me, that milk was a problem. It was like an Ex-Lax to him. His wife was in the hospital. I couldn't ask her. I tell you, if you can work one-on-one, minute by minute, day by day, all day long, or all night long, you will learn, the hard way, but you'll definitely get the idea.

Well, let me tell you about another situation in the bathroom. We have those that we call the hand washers. Oh, that sounds easy enough. Go in the bathroom, cut on the water and wash your hands. Well, it doesn't work that way. These are the people that go into the bathroom and sit on the toilet and use one square of paper to wipe themselves four or five times. The instant that they get up, they turn around and wash their hands in the toilet water. Now they are coming out and they are shaking their hands. "Oh no!" It's a shock when you find out that everything they put in the toilet is still there, and they washed their hands in the mess.

NOW THAT'S A LITTLE SHOCKER

I think for the people that wash their hands in the toilet, they don't understand or they don't remember that they could cut the faucet on in the sink and wash their hands. They find it easier to turn around, see this big white bowl with a little something in it, and wash their hands in it. Now, they wouldn't be a patient or at least an Alzheimer's one if they knew how to go in there, use the toilet, wipe themselves with plenty of paper, cut the faucet on, get a little bit of soap, wash their hands, get a paper towel, and dry, and then come on back out. I wouldn't be telling you these stories. That's why you actually have to watch and learn and find out what it is that Alzheimer's patients are all about.

I haven't told you about the strippers. These are the nice people. They go to the bathroom, use the toilet, never wash their hands, but every time they come out, half of them are naked. If they're not all naked, their underwear is gone. You go into the bathroom and look for the underwear. You might find it underneath the toilet, underneath the tub, stuck up in the corner with the toilet paper, folded up, or put up on the shelf with the towels you just washed. These are the strippers.

What about those king-sized babies? I'm talking about

the patient that you take in the bathroom and sometimes you need two or three people to help you get a diaper off of them. Just imagine, one person holding their hands, the other person taking off the diaper, and the other person cleaning their butt. Well, what happens to that person when the diaper is off and they decide to stand there and poop right in the palm of your hands? Well, you have just about blown your stack. You don't know if you are going or coming and you say, "This is it, no more. I just can't stand it." Well, don't feel bad. It's going to happen tomorrow and the next day, and the day after. You know what makes it all worthwhile? When you finish that patient and he or she looks at you with this sad face and mumbles a few words saying, "Thank you".

GUILT

This is Connie, just coming back from a support group for Alzheimer's disease. The topic for today was guilt. I found a lot of people have guilt, even to the point where they need a support group to help them realize that what they do for their parents, sister, brother and anyone else is okay. It's just nobody's willing to say to them, "It's okay." They use the support groups to discuss a variety of topics until they feel satisfied that what they did was "okay." They have tried everything they can to take care of their love ones, but sometimes that's just not enough. When they are 60 and 70 years old themselves, it's hard taking care of an 80 or 90 year old. They're all in bad health. Sometimes they need the support of other people just like them, in the same situations, some worse than others, to say, "I wish I had the strength you did to put your mother away." I hear people tell me all the time, "I visit my mother everyday at the nursing home." It's only guilt. Mom's being taken care of 24 hours a day and you are home worrying yourself to death. If we could take guilt out of our everyday living, maybe we could live a little longer.

Guilt is a funny emotion that humans have. You know you go through your life feeling guilty about everything.

Did I raise the children right? Was I a good wife? Am I a good coworker? You know, guilt wears on you. It wears and tears on the body when you're dealing with a family member that has some type of illness, not necessarily Alzheimer's, but just about any kind of disease or disabling sickness. A person feels guilty because they can walk, talk, and hold a spoon in their hand.

I was listening to a lady at the support group this morning and she was telling us about the guilt trip she was on. She had her gallbladder removed and then the doctor told her that everything was okay. Well, she thought that the gallbladder was her punishment and that is why it was removed. That was guilt. She thought she was perfect. She wanted to take care of her mother the right way, and no one else could do it better than she could. You know guilt can kill. When your mother goes back to her childhood and she's no longer married to your father, she wants to go home to her mother. Her name is not Smith anymore but she's back to her maiden name. It could be Jones or Steward or Matthew or something else. Then you have that guilt that my mother is my child and I'm the mother. Then the guilt steps in again and you know that you have to switch roles. If you don't make that switch and take over, and get things in order, guilt will eat you alive.

I find that guilt is even harder on the man. If his wife has something like Alzheimer's disease or dementia and he finds that she is no longer his wife and don't remember him, it will make him feel pretty bad. He won't know which way is up. Then guilt steps in again and he says, "Oh, Lord, what can I do? How can I help her?" You don't find any answers at home. You go out looking for a support group to get some answers or ideas on the type of care that she requires, and maybe it could help you in the long run.

You know, I find that children of the sick and elderly have bigger problems than their fathers and mothers; guilt! They now have to be their mother's mother or their father's father and they're totally upset. They find themselves saying, "Little girl, sit down. Little girl, get up. Little girl, get dressed. Little girl, eat your food. It's good for you." Now the family is really unorganized.

The really scary part comes when a mother, father, or sister says, "Who are you? Are you my cousin? Are you my uncle? That's really scary. You know who you are, but they don't know. There's no convincing them. By telling them, "I'm your daughter, Mom" and "I'm your son, Dad," it doesn't work that way. Everybody is confused and then there's your guilt because you are saying but "Mom, I'm going to help take care of you." You say, "Oh mom, please, it's just me. It's Bernadette or it's Stephanie or it's Roxanne." Then she says, "You're lying, you aren't my child. You're nobody."

The scariest part is when they say, "I'm not married." I don't have any children. I'm only 12. I want to go home to my mother." Or they tell the sons, "Oh no, don't take off my clothes. It's personal. You can't do that. Lady's don't undress in front of men. Please stop, stop." Then the son just dies of shame. Then, there's guilt again. Then he says, "Lord, somebody needs to help me. I can't do it alone." Now, you're looking for a support group or you're looking for some professional help. You need someone to tell you in which direction you should go. How can I help my mother without her thinking I'm a stranger."

Now you're at your wit's end and you want to go to the library. You want to look up the book on Alzheimer disease. You want to see what they wrote about people with Alzheimer's. These books can tell you a little about real life, the one-on-one, and the everyday living. What you are doing in your home, with your mother, your father, your sister, or your brother? Nobody wants to write about that. You know exactly what you have to do. You have to stop, step back, look at the situation, think about your mom, your dad, or your sister, and the type of person that they were before they got sick. What would they allow? What would they disallow? Think about that as a tool. That tool is the lifestyle they lived, and you can use it on them. If they dislike this, or they don't want to dress like that, or they won't eat this, or they won't say that, that's the tools you start off with. You still have to go out and do some research, go to support groups, and even ask families just like yours, with situations like yours, for some answers until you find some way to work with your family member. If you don't ask, you'll feel like you're in prison, and if you're in prison, you'll be burned out. If you get burned out, you'll be in the hospital and mom or dad and your sister will be still home getting on someone else's nerves. You won't let that happen. You won't let your mom or sister or dad get on someone else's nerves, because you figure if mom can take care of 13 children, why can't one or two or three take care of mom. Whether you know it or not, there aren't any books on parenting and there aren't any on one-on-one Alzheimer's treatments in the home. You learn it day by day, inch by inch, minute by minute, and if you're lucky, you can find some one that might give

What You Hear Is Not What You See

you a clue.

You know people with Alzheimer's can be very quiet or sometime combative. They don't always know exactly what they're doing. I hear family members tell us that their mom is leaving the house and going to church. "Mom has no feelings for me. My Mom doesn't know me." I hear husbands say, "My wife doesn't love me anymore, he would continue, 'My wife doesn't know who I am anymore. Then I'm truly upset. What do I do? How can I prove to her I'm her husband? I married her 30 years ago. I'm 50 and my mother doesn't know that I am her daughter. To her I could be the next door neighbor.'" Sometimes, somewhere a glimmer of light goes off and Mom looks at you, a spark will come between you two, and Mom will say, "Mary is that you?"

You know, it's not all bad because they're sick. It's not all the time that they don't know you and it's not all the time that they don't want you to touch them. For all the work you do for them, there is a moment where Mom will say, "Are you my daughter, then another question, 'Are you my husband?'" She would pause, "I used to have six or seven children. 'I don't know where they are now.' 'I used to have a husband.' 'I don't know where he is now.'" You could be standing right there, but just for her to even recognize you for a minute has made your day, your year, and the guilt that you felt is gone. For all the love you wanted to give back to your Mom, you can give it to her just for one moment, and that makes everything that you do and everything that you have felt and suffered okay.

These are some of the things that happen in family life everyday when you're dealing with guilt. I had a patient at one time, but the daughter was the "real" patient. It's a terrible thing to watch this disease eat my mother alive," she would say. To me, I feel like this is a living death, and I am in virtual grief. The lady also told me that she could run a big business and she could handle a staff of 50, but when it came to her mother, one little 90 year old lady, weighing about 60 pounds, she couldn't tell you how to take care of her; but I knew. I would go to her house and visit her on my day off. Just knowing that this lady could run her own business, I would tell her what she could do for your mother. In other words, on her job she was the boss, but in her house she was still the child and she refused to make that switch. For her, and in her lifetime, it made the job of taking care of her mother her first priority. She lived in an awful lot of guilt. If she couldn't teach herself how to take care of her mother, she thought that she would end up like her; her children and grandchildren would have to take care of her. She knew her mother. I think she would put herself in a nursing home if she could, because she couldn't call herself a caregiver; she really wasn't. She was still a child that lived in the house under her sick mother. A caregiver is a person that has knowledge of the person that they're caring for. You have to do research. You have to get out there, whether it hurts you or not. You have to find out the "best way" to take care of your mother. It's very important that you ask questions. It's a dumb person or a hurting person that never asks questions. You have to learn, and I mean learn as if you were back in school. You have to learn how to deal with different situations as they arise. If you don't, you'll be caught in a web like a spider and the fly.

DO YOU KNOW?

Do you know - That some of them can't tell if you are a man or a woman.

Do you know - That they can sing all of the songs from the 40s and 50s.

Do you know - They know their feet hurt but not know it's because their shoes are on the wrong foot.

Do you know - That they can eat paper tissues all day and never swallow them.

Do you know - That sex is at the top of their list.

Do you know - That they can show you love, from a punch in your face, to shifting in their clothes, to just smiling.

Do you know - That most of the men still want to go to work and still have a wife.

Do you know - That if a client thinks you are some family member that they like, you can't change their mind.

Do you know - That they call on the Lord just to make a bowel movement.

Do you know - That if a client carries money in his or her pockets, he or she will catch a taxi.

Do you know - That a female client, in a kitchen, will try and kill you with a knife. Do you know - That a client will take ten different pills, get sick and won't know what caused it.

Do you know - That if a client answers questions that they don't know, they will say something ridiculous.

Do you know - That a client will put Sweet and Low, paste, salt, or juice on food and think it tastes good.

Do you know - That a client will put coffee in his or her cereal and think it's okay.

Do you know - That a client can get mad at you for no reason at all, and if you call on a dead family member, it would make them react or calm down.

Do you know - That a client can wet their clothes or defecate in their pants and then want to know who did it, thinking that they didn't.

Do you know — The caregiver that thinks they know everything about nursing only cares for their own family members. Well I'm here to tell you just let me do my job of 30 years. I am tired of people talking to us as if we are dummies. You tell us how to put a diaper on your mother or husband. You tell us how many times he or she should go to the toilet, what to eat, or what not to eat. Just because you pay us, it doesn't give you the right to abuse us with your smart words. I want to tell some of you caregivers that are really the wives, daughters and sons, that you only have six months to one year experience working with patients that are unpredictable in behavior and speech. Well, I can tell you, I know them better then you because I do the one-on-one eight days a week and thirty hours a day. I know them inside and out. Just let me do my job. Let me help you get through one day at a time. I was trained for many years for this job, and I do it well. If you let me give you some tips on nursing care, you wouldn't be as nasty or burned out as you are.

Do you know - Just because they stop talking, walking, sleeping and eating, they are not dead nor are they just a vegetable, lying around doing nothing. This is my classroom. This is where years of learning and teaching comes into play. If you could look through a looking glass, you would be surprised at what's still in the minds of patients. All is not lost! With my training, I can hold onto the mind a little longer; if you just let me do my job.

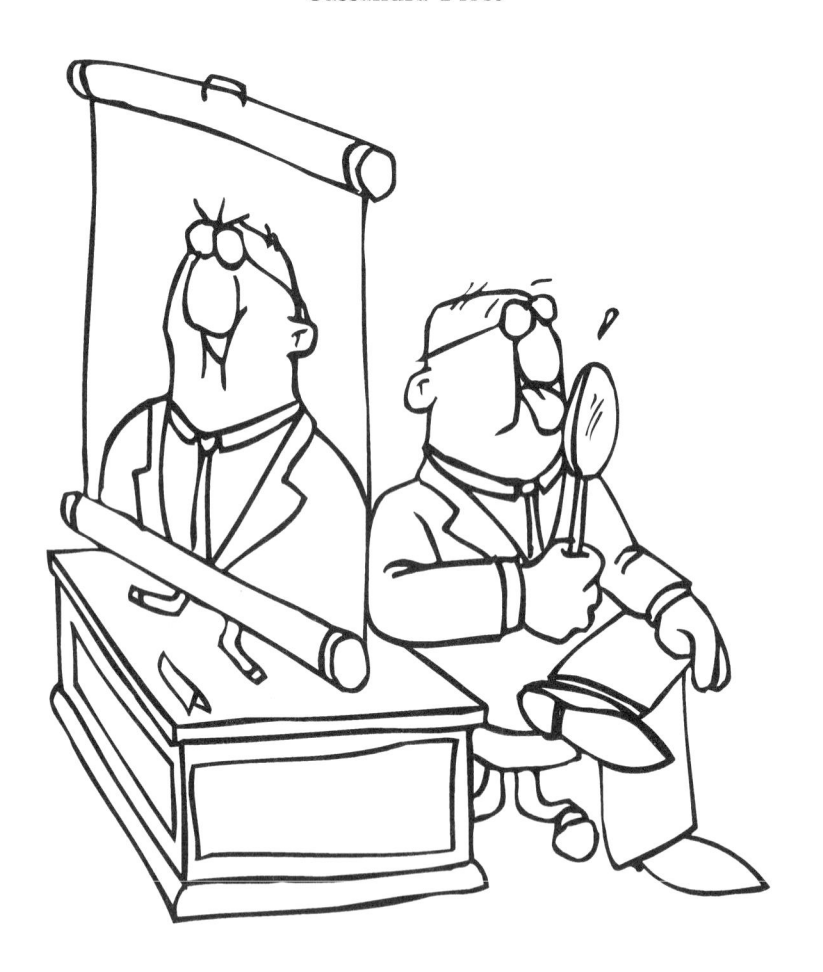

Man in the Mirror

Bill

"Who are the people in the mirror?"

"No, that's a fat man."

Connie

"It's you."

"It's Bill."

What You Hear Is Not What You See

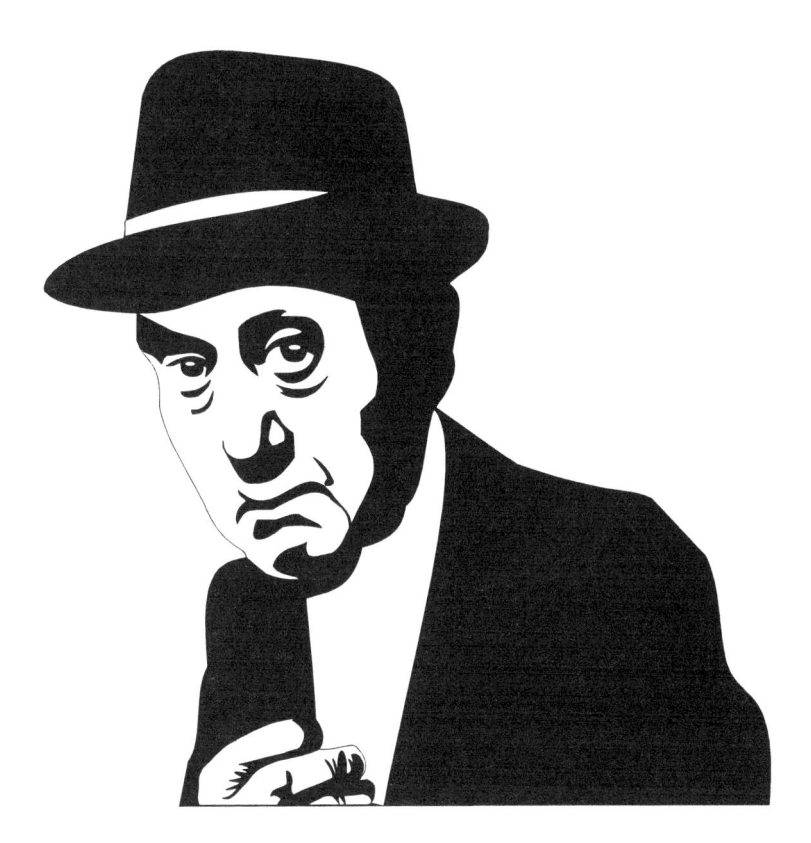

Birthday

Connie

"Happy Birthday."

Bill

"It's not my birthday, not until 1929."

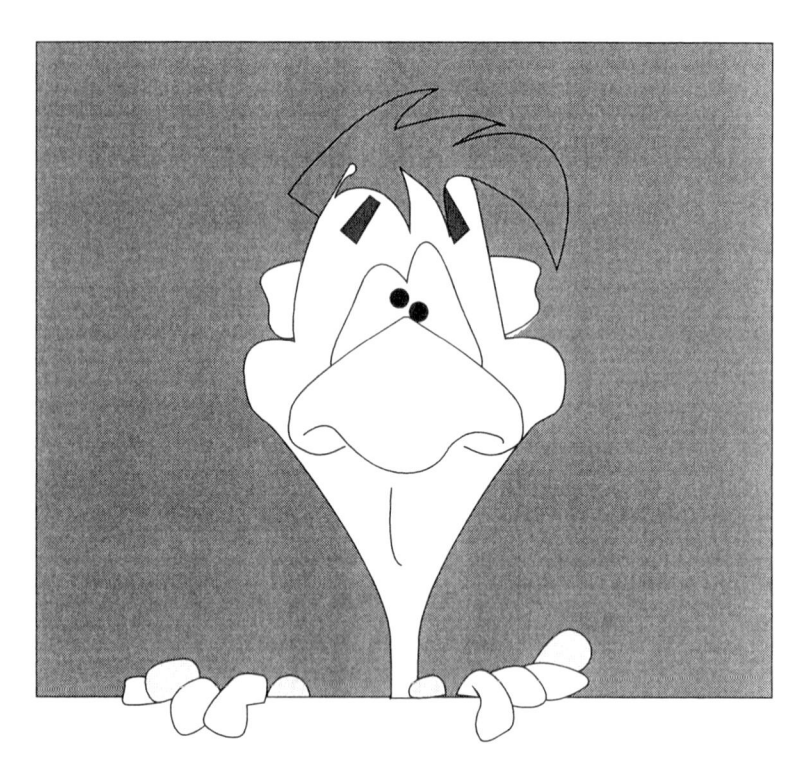

"Who is a frog's natural enemy?"

"Snakes and the devil."

What You Hear Is Not What You See

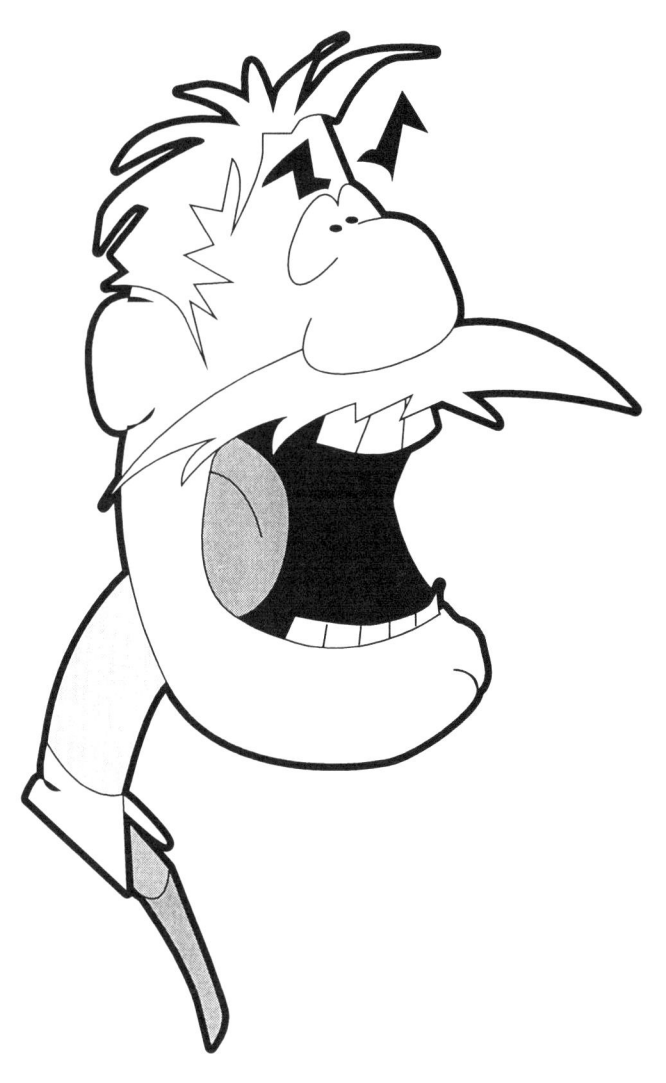

If I've just eaten and tell you that I'm hungry,

it's OK.

Just feed me.

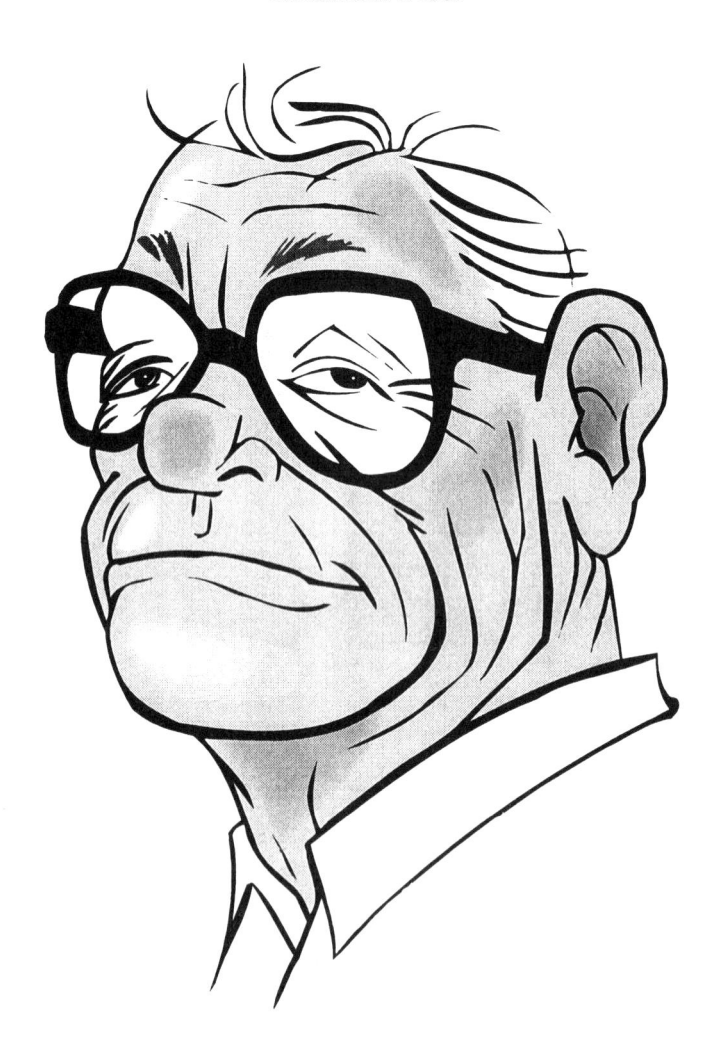

If I look confused,

it's OK.

I don't know it.

What You Hear Is Not What You See

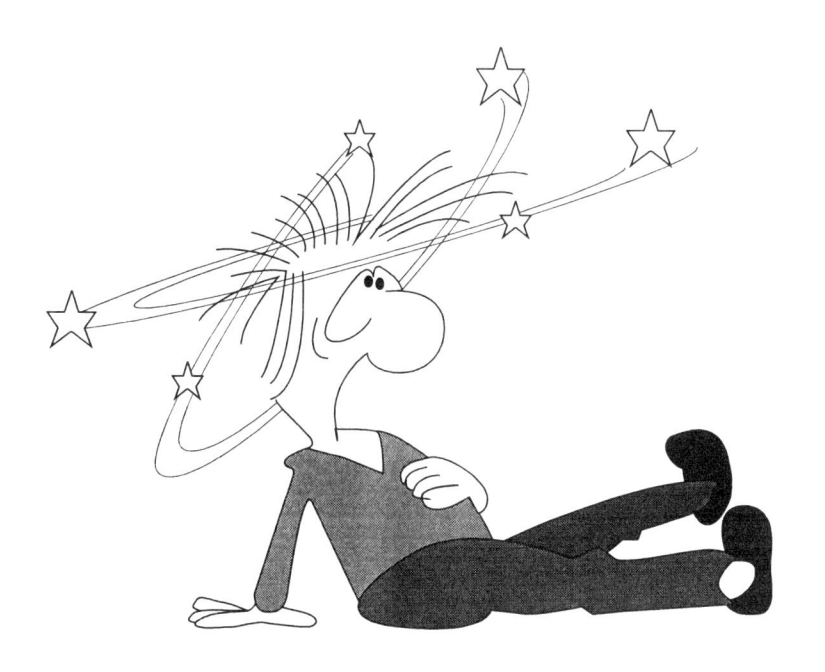

If I forget who you are, just say it a couple hundred times.

I might get it.

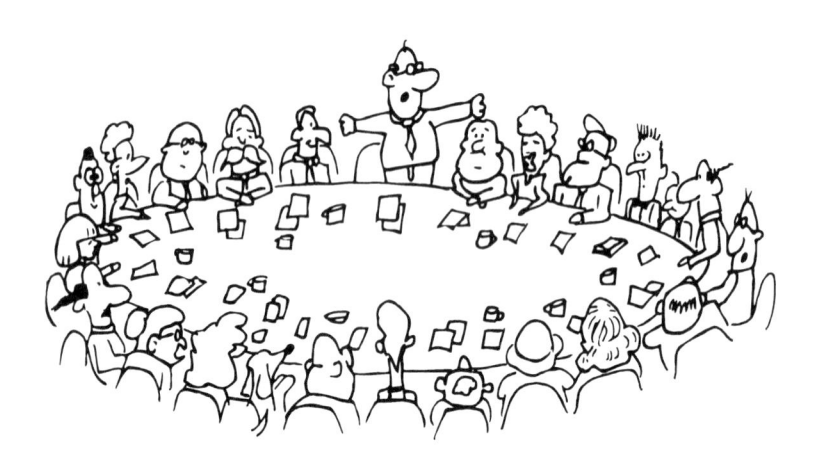

If I see all my childhood friends and most of them are dead,

it's OK.

They can't hurt you.

What You Hear Is Not What You See

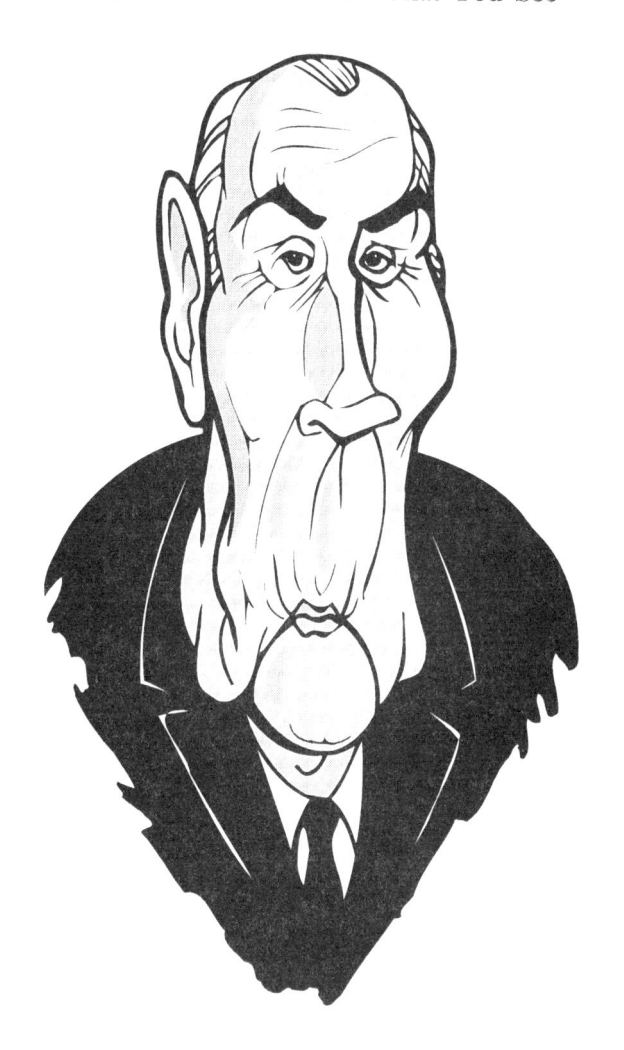

If I see all my childhood friends and most of them are dead,

it's OK.

Just say hi.

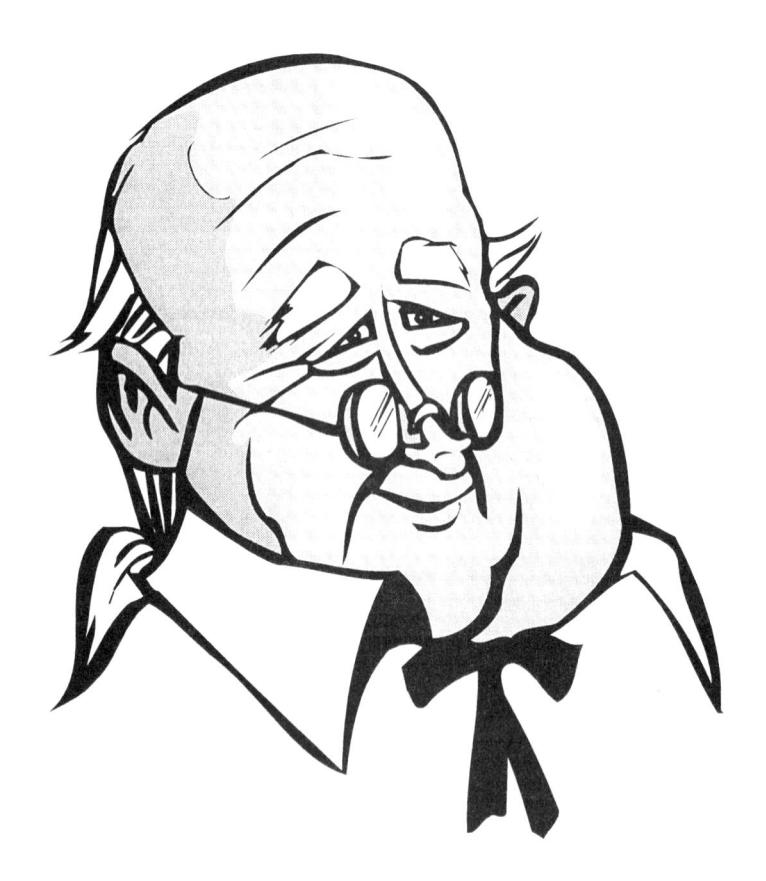

If my kids are now my old buddies,

it's OK.

Just give me a beer and let's talk about the good old days.

What You Hear Is Not What You See

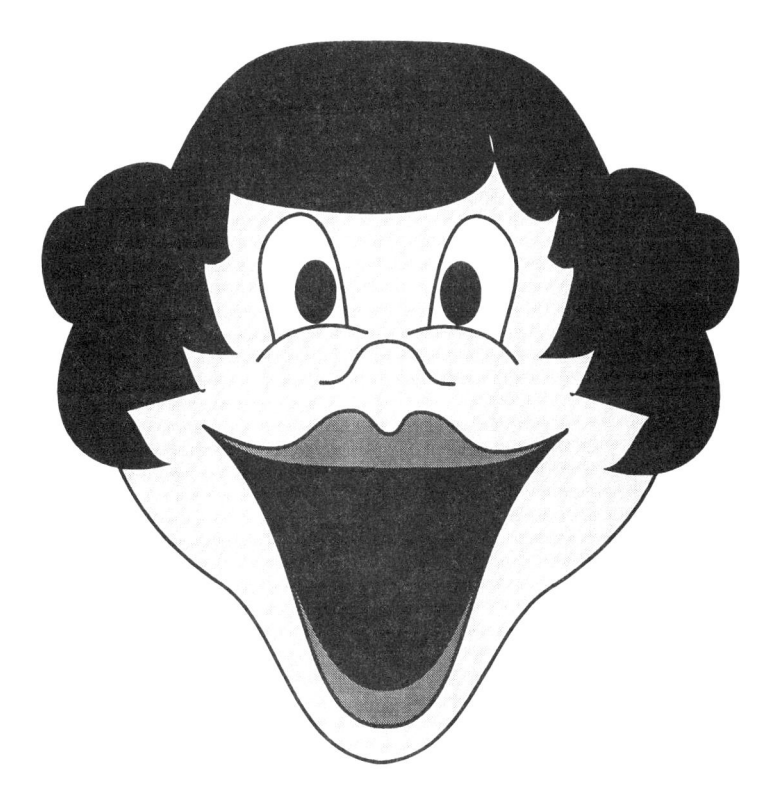

If I talk normal,

it's OK.

Don't believe anything I say.

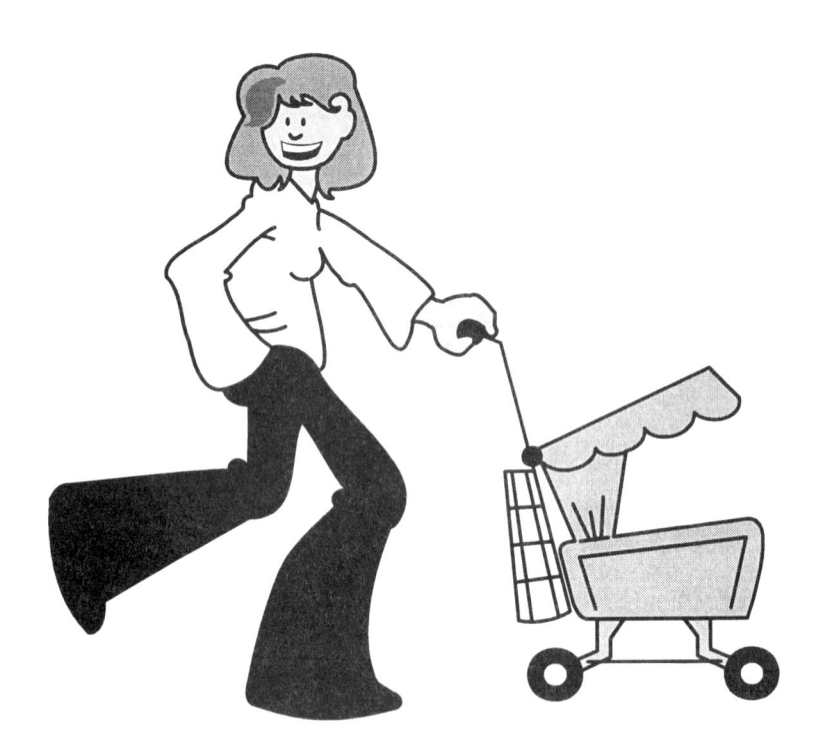

If I tell you I can drive,

it's OK.

Hide the key!

What You Hear Is Not What You See

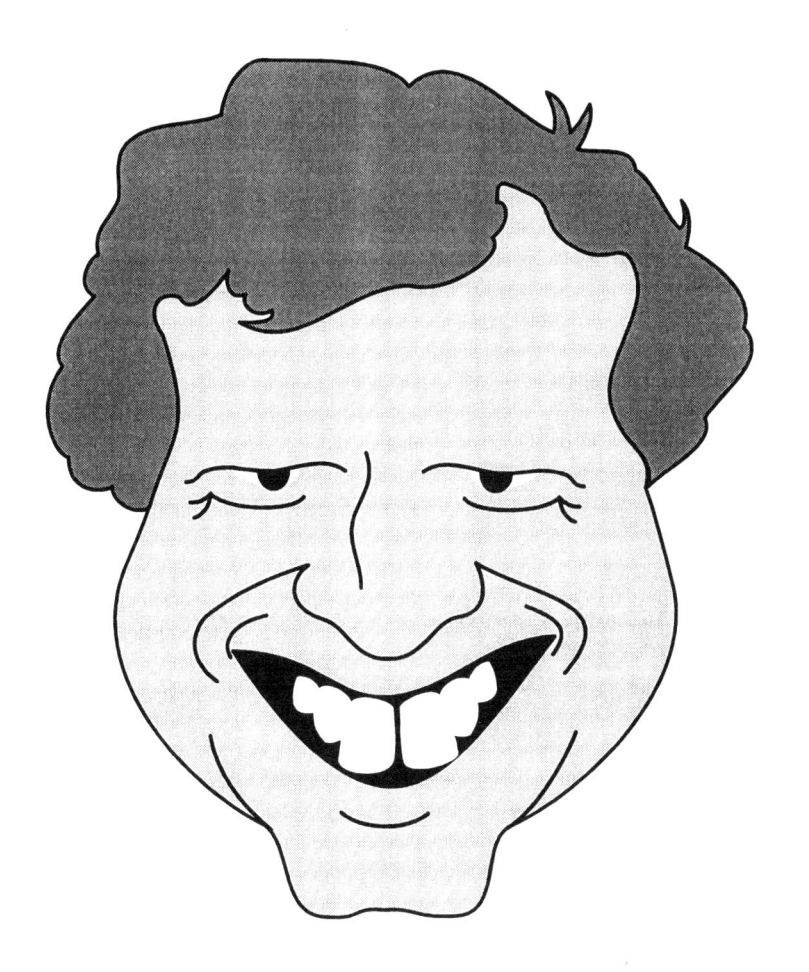

If I tell you that I'm leaving,

it's OK.

Believe it!

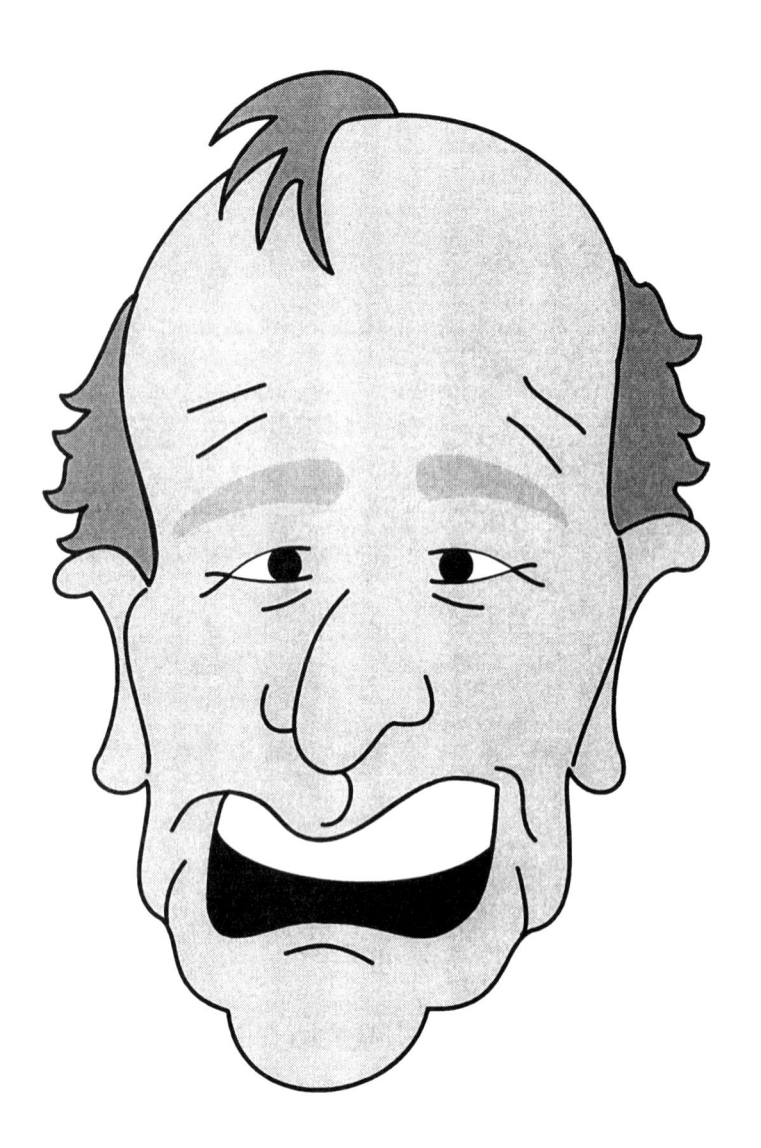

If I look confused,

it's OK.

I'm thinking of nothing.